ULCERATIVE COLITIS

CLINICAL GASTROENTEROLOGY MONOGRAPH SERIES
John M. Dietschy, M.D., *Series Editor*

Gastrointestinal Bleeding: Diagnosis and Management
John A. Balint, M.B., F.R.C.P.
I. James Sarfeh, M.D.
Martin B. Fried, M.D.

Complications of Gastric Surgery
David Fromm, M.D.

Diseases of the Gallbladder and Biliary System
Leslie J. Schoenfield, M.D.

Ulcerative Colitis
Michael J. Goodman, B.M., B.Ch., D.Phil., M.R.C.P.
Marshall Sparberg, M.D., F.A.C.P.

Viral Hepatitis
Raymond S. Koff, M.D.

ULCERATIVE COLITIS

MICHAEL J. GOODMAN, B.M., B.Ch., D.Phil., M.R.C.P.
Consultant Physician and Gastroenterologist,
Bury General Hospital, Greater Manchester, England;
Formerly Assistant Professor of Medicine,
University of Chicago, Chicago, Illinois

MARSHALL SPARBERG, M.D., F.A.C.P.
Associate Professor of Medicine,
Northwestern University, Chicago, Illinois

Foreword by
JOSEPH B. KIRSNER, M.D., Ph.D., M.A.C.P.
Louis Block Distinguished Service Professor of Medicine,
University of Chicago, Chicago, Illinois

A Wiley Medical Publication
John Wiley & Sons
New York • Chichester • Brisbane • Toronto

Library of Congress Cataloging in Publication Data:

Goodman, Michael John, 1944-
Ulcerative colitis.

(Clinical gastroenterology monograph series)
Includes bibliographical references and index.
1. Ulcerative colitis. I. Sparberg, Marshall,
1936– joint author. II. Title. III. Series.
[DNLM: 1. Colitis, Ulcerative. WI522 G653u]
RC862.C63G66 616.3'44 78-8686
ISBN 0-471-48895-X

Printed in the United States of America

10 9 8 7 6 5 4 3 2 1

FOREWORD

Not too long ago the "nonspecific" inflammatory bowel diseases (IBD), ulcerative colitis and Crohn's disease, were regarded as unusual, relatively uncommon entities, of interest exclusively to a few gastroenterologists. The situation today is much different. Ulcerative colitis and Crohn's disease are far more common today than in years past, and they are increasing in frequency, especially Crohn's disease. The estimated numbers of IBD patients in the United States alone exceed 500,000 people, and the figures continue to increase.

Though more than 100 years have elapsed since the initial description of ulcerative colitis by Wilks, virtually every aspect of this disease—etiology, recurrent course, complications and therapy—remains obscure. Because of the intriguing nature of the bowel disease per se, and also because of the interesting associated complications, few human illnesses, including the once "glamorous" connective tissue disorders, offer as many investigative opportunities. Indeed, ulcerative colitis (and Crohn's disease) have emerged as one of the Rosetta stones of modern medicine in highlighting the scope of the gastrointestinal, cellular, and immune responses to disease, and the biologic nature of the many bowel-related local and systemic problems.

The epidemiology of IBD is intriguing. Ulcerative colitis is worldwide in its distribution, with substantial, but unexplained, geographic variations in severity and course (e.g., it is unheard of in mainland China, infrequent in South America, mild in Japan, and severe in the United States). Ulcerative colitis (and Crohn's disease) has been reported from more than 50 countries in all continents of the globe. The similar clinical features and course of IBD everywhere in the world, despite different ethnic populations, sociocultural customs and dietary habits, also are noteworthy. Though the precise incidence is not known, ulcerative colitis appears to be leveling off in recent years, in contrast to Crohn's disease, which is increasing steadily everywhere. Yet ulcerative colitis patients at present comprise 50 to 60% of all IBD patients seen at major medical centers. Ulcerative colitis is much more common among white people and probably more common among Jewish people; but all ethnic groups are affected. The frequency of ulcerative colitis among children, adolescents, and young adults always has been a curious demographic feature, probably of pathogenetic importance; though no age group is exempt, including infants. Since amebic colitis and lymphopathia venereum, among other specific entities, with new knowledge, were separated from the originally broad category of "nonspecific" ulcerative colitis group, and since a "nonspecific proctitis" is observed not infrequently in people proctoscoped for diarrhea, the possibility remains of other "specific" forms of colitis within the heterogeneous parent group.

The etiological theories, attributed to most chronic diseases of unknown cause (bacteria, viruses, psychogenic or immunologic abnormalities), have been applied to ulcerative colitis without success. The cause or causes remain unknown, and the possible etiological interrelationship between ulcerative colitis and Crohn's disease remains as speculative today as in the past. The microbiological possibilities of earlier years (diplostreptococcus, spherophorus necrophorus, *Entamoeba histolytica,* bacillary dysentery, etc.) have been supplanted by interest in pathogenic coliform organisms, bacteroides, pseudomonas-like organisms, other anaerobes, and enteric viruses. The possibility of an earlier antecedent infection of the bowel, or perhaps an antibiotic-mediated change in the bacterial flora of the bowel, "setting the stage" for the later development of colitis has long been an attractive hypothesis; especially because bacteria, bacterial endotoxins, and metabolic products somehow must be involved in the etiology and pathogenesis. However, knowledge of the aerobic and anaerobic flora of the gut in IBD, the possible actions of aerobic and anaerobic bacterial endotoxins and metabolites upon the bowel wall and upon immunologically mediated gut reactions, remains limited.

The role of psychogenic difficulties in the pathogenesis of ulcerative colitis remains anecdotal and debatable. The central nervous system, of course, is a key regulator of gastrointestinal function and gastrointestinal integrity. The chronological association between the onset, the recurrences, and the severity of ulcerative colitis and individually significant emotional events, remains unchallenged. However, the psychoanalytically oriented concepts of the 1930s and 1940s have lost appeal as a clarifying hypothesis, because of insufficient evidence and because the psychoanalytical approach has not proved adequate for either control or cure of the disease. Controlled studies actually have revealed significant emotional difficulties more often among patients with the irritable bowel syndrome than among patients with ulcerative colitis. Nevertheless, psychogenic influences undoubtedly play a role in the evolution of ulcerative colitis; a relationship awaiting clarification of the biological impact of emotional disorders upon gastrointestinal function. The renewed emphasis upon an individual failure of adaptive responses to stress may provide useful information, especially if such studies include objective measurements of physiological, biochemical and intracellular events in the gut in relation to the stressful events. The recently discovered peptidergic neuroses in the small and the large intestine, and in the brain, offer yet another exciting new approach toward clarifying the relationship between the central nervous system and the gastrointestinal tract.

The possible involvement of immunological mechanisms in ulcerative colitis, first proposed by Kirsner and Palmer in 1954, continues to generate important observations. Indeed, the impact of this concept has far exceeded the original application to inflammatory bowel disease. A large number of significant projects related directly to the gastrointestinal response to disease has been initiated. Thus, immunological studies have demonstrated the central role of the gastrointestinal tract in the immunological homeostasis of the body, the integrative function, of T- and B- lymphocytes, and the gut-associated lymphoid tissue, local events in the development of gastrointestinal immunologically mediated responses to IBD, and the locally protective role of secretory IgA at the gastrointestinal epithelial surface. As in all other areas of medical science, new knowledge generates new questions. In ulcerative colitis, more information is needed on gastrointestinal immune responses generally, the local gastrointestinal antibody system, the functions of the gastrointestinal lymphoid tissue, the role of other cellular components of the IBD tissue reaction (polymorphonuclear cells, eosinophils, basophils), the possible role of the complement system in the IBD process, the effects of various bacteria and their metabolic products, and the facts involved in bacterial adherence and non-adherence to bowel epithelium, among other problems.

The concept of an individual vulnerability and perhaps also individual resistance to ulcerative colitis, also proposed by Kirsner and Palmer in 1954, thus far has yielded a limited number of studies. However, the hypothesis is even more attractive today, in view of the rising number of familial occurrences of IBD, and because of new knowledge of host defense mechanisms and of genetic influences in human disease. An important potential source of new information in this area relates to histocompatibility haplotypes and their relationship to genetically influenced immune mechanisms, and to possible deficiencies in the complement system. While no specific haplotype has yet been identified for ulcerative colitis not complicated by ankylosing spondylitis or iritis, present knowledge in this area is limited and further study may disclose a significant relationship to a particular histocompatibility haplotype. Familial IBD begins at an earlier age and tends to be more complicated than usual. This particular group of patients, therefore, deserves intensive study of genetic and other influences as a likely source of important information on the pathogenesis of ulcerative colitis.

As intriguing as are these etiological possibilities, the clinical problems of accurate evaluation and effective management of the patient with ulcerative colitis are even more compelling at the present time. Those who have not had the responsibility for the care of the sick person, child or young adult, afflicted with a chronic recurrent disease of obscure origin, often requiring surgery, capable of causing many complications, prolonged invalidism and even death, together with emotional, social and economic devastation for the patient and the family, cannot fully appreciate the urgent need for better understanding and more effective treatment of IBD. Ulcerative colitis, in fact, can be as incapacitating as chronic renal insufficiency, as relentless as leukemia, and as malignant as any neoplasm. Surprisingly, in the late 1970s, there continues to be only limited awareness of the "global" nature of IBD and of the need for comprehensive evaluation of the patient as a basis for continuously effective therapy. All too often, patients are "treated" with large quantities of steroids and/or sulfasalazine, without consideration of the nutritional and emotional status of the patient, without awareness of the many details of symptomatic care helpful in reducing the need for hazardous drugs, and without recognition of the importance of continuing control of the disease.

For, despite the limitations in our knowledge, ulcerative colitis can often be controlled with a comprehensive, individualized program. The "therapeutic philosophies" of physicians who deal with IBD chronometrically, i.e., on the basis of "recovery either within seven to ten days of initial treatment or else surgery," or of the physician who delegates the IBD problem to a psychiatrist without careful review of the clinical situation and without adequate medical care, are unacceptable. Patience, hope, perseverance, interest in the patient, and attention to details by the skilled and humane physician are important ingredients of successful medical treatment; controlled studies or not. And, in those patients requiring surgical treatment because of complications or irreversible damage to the bowel, the conditions for operation, selection of the appropriate procedure, and details of postoperative management, and subsequent rehabilitation also require an informed and experienced approach.

It is in these clinical aspects of ulcerative colitis that my recent colleagues, Michael Goodman and Marshall Sparberg, have made a notable contribution. The major purpose of this monograph has been to provide the general internist and the primary care physician, who are often the initial medical contact for the IBD patient, with clear, practical guidelines as to the clinical nature of ulcerative colitis, the accurate differential diagnosis, and the associated clinical problems. The concise recommendations for the evaluation of the patient, the appropriate use of diagnostic resources, the treatment of various complications, including the early detection of colonic cancer, the follow-up observations, the details of surgical treatment, preoperative and postoperative care, and ileostomy care, followed by sections on ulcerative colitis in childhood, ulcerative colitis in pregnancy, and a concluding chapter on prognosis complete a comprehensive and practical approach to ulcerative colitis which will be useful to all physicians.

This book will be helpful, therefore, not only to the primary care physician and the general internist, but also to the gastroenterologic consultant who often assumes continuing responsibility for the care of the patient, and to the gastrointestinal surgeon involved in the operative management of this disorder. This book will facilitate the orderly and thorough approach to the IBD patient, which is important not only in the management of the problem but also in generating useful new ideas on the disorder itself. Thoughtful scrutiny of the clinical course, leading to perceptive clinical studies, in association with imaginative research by resourceful investigators, remains the chief hope for revealing the secrets of ulcerative colitis, as did the Rosetta stone in unlocking the secrets of Egyptian civilization several thousand years ago.

Joseph B. Kirsner, M.D., Ph.D., M.A.C.P.

SERIES PREFACE

During the past decade remarkable progress has been made in our understanding of many basic physiological processes related to liver and gastrointestinal tract functions. Much of this information has led to significant improvements in our understanding of clinical diseases that alter normal hepatic and intestinal function and in the therapy of these diseases. Innumerable examples can be cited. For instance, the application of basic principles of physical chemistry has clarified considerably the manner in which cholesterol is solubilized in bile. Related studies have identified the causes of cholesterol gallstones in several large groups of patients, and specific forms of therapy for the prevention or the dissolution of such stones are now available. Other experimental work that relies heavily on basic techniques of immunology and electron microscopy has identified specific infectious agents affecting liver function. These studies, in turn, have provided considerable insight into the different clinical syndromes included under the general heading of viral hepatitis, raising the possibility that effective immunization against these organisms may soon be available. Equally impressive advances have been made in our understanding of the control of gastric secretion and peptic ulcer disease, in the causes of intestinal malabsorption, and in radiographic and endoscopic methods for examining the liver and gastrointestinal tract.

This explosion of knowledge in gastroenterology poses a particularly difficult problem for those interested in the dissemination of new medical information to students, house officers, and medical practitioners. Often advances have come so quickly that the information presented in standard textbooks is outdated before the books become available. Also, it is difficult to revise such texts rapidly because of the large number of authors involved and the long production time necessary for these books. Finally, the space available to authors for extensively reviewing both the basic physiological concepts and their clinical implications is limited in most texts and in more rapidly published medical journals.

This series of volumes published under the general title "Clinical Gastroenterology Monograph" was conceived and designed to overcome many of these difficulties and to bring to the medical practitioner the most current information on the pathophysiology and treatment of major areas of disease affecting the liver and gastrointestinal tract. Each volume covers an important group of related disorders and is sufficiently long to allow for extensive discussion of their basic pathophysiological, clinical, and therapeutic aspects. New volumes will appear regularly, and a special effort will be made to identify areas for inclusion in the series in which there is a rapidly expanding body of information relevant to the care of patients with a particular gastrointestinal disorder. Existing volumes will be updated and republished frequently where continued advances in information justify such rapid revision.

It is hoped that this series will provide a continuously evolving and current reference source for the broad spectrum of physicians who deal with patients with diseases of the liver and gastrointestinal tract.

John M. Dietschy, M.D.

PREFACE

This book has been written for the general internist who is called upon to treat patients with ulcerative colitis, rather than primarily for the specialist gastroenterologist, although we would hope that gastroenterologists would find many helpful points in the book. The general surgeon, too, is frequently involved in the care of such patients, and we hope that this book will be valuable to him also. It is not designed to be an exhaustive text on ulcerative colitis, but rather a handbook for the management of patients with this disease. We have inserted references only to illustrate and justify points we have made and to provide sources for the further study of particular aspects about which the reader may wish to have more detail.

For the sake of brevity, we have used "he," "him," and "his" in referring to patients and physicians, not to exclude female patients or female physicians, nor as a snub to feminists, but simply as a convention in the absence of a satisfactory term for "he or she." Throughout the book, we have used "sigmoidoscopy" instead of "protoscopy," the "irritable colon syndrome" rather than "spastic colon" or the "irritable bowel syndrome," and "Crohn's disease" rather than "regional enteritis" or "granulomatous colitis."

We should like to acknowledge our colleagues Drs. A. L. Baker, M. O. Blackstone, Paul Frank, D. J. O'Connell, R. H. Riddell, and K. Soltani for lending us photographs for the illustrations, and Dr. A. R. Moossa for advice on the details of the preparation of patients for surgery. Figures 2.1 and 20.1 are reproduced by kind permission of their original authors and publishers. One of us (M.J.G.) would like to acknowledge the Gastro-Intestinal Research Foundation of Chicago for salary support during the writing of this book.

Finally, but foremost, we should like to express our warmest gratitude to our teachers, Dr. Joseph B. Kirsner and Dr. Sidney Truelove, for teaching us much of what we know about ulcerative colitis and much of what is written in this book.

MICHAEL J. GOODMAN
MARSHALL SPARBERG

CONTENTS

I. THE NATURE OF ULCERATIVE COLITIS
1. What is Ulcerative Colitis? 3
2. Epidemiology 6
3. Etiology 11
4. Pathology 16

II. THE CLINICAL PRESENTATION
5. Symptoms 31
6. Physical Signs 37
7. Local Complications 41
8. Systemic Complications 50

III. THE DIAGNOSIS
9. Differential Diagnosis 67
10. Evaluation of the Patient 75
11. Endoscopy and Biopsy 77
12. Radiology 89

IV. MANAGEMENT
13. Medical Treatment 109
14. Treatment of Complications 138
15. Follow-Up 144
16. Surgical Treatment 148
17. Ileostomy Care 160
18. Ulcerative Colitis in Childhood 169
19. Ulcerative Colitis and Pregnancy 173

V. THE NATURAL HISTORY
20. Prognosis 183

References 193
Index 199

ULCERATIVE COLITIS

I

The Nature of Ulcerative Colitis

1

WHAT IS ULCERATIVE COLITIS?

Ulcerative colitis is a chronic inflammatory disease of the large intestine of unknown etiology. In its acute stages it resembles an infectious disease, but no microorganism has been definitely established as its cause. It can be defined according to its pathological features, which give rise to typical endoscopic (sigmoidoscopic and colonoscopic) and radiological appearances. Current theories of the etiology will be discussed in Chapter 3, the pathological features in Chapter 4, the endoscopic appearances in Chapter 11, and the radiological features in Chapter 12.

DIAGNOSIS

The firmest diagnosis of ulcerative colitis can be made following a total proctocolectomy operation, when the entire colon and rectum are available for a full pathological examination. Otherwise, and most often, the diagnosis is made from endoscopic, radiological, and biopsy evidence obtained from patients with suggestive symptoms. Such evidence may be incomplete to a certain extent; and in arriving at the diagnosis, it is helpful to exclude other conditions in which the colonic mucosa can be inflamed. These conditions include infectious diseases, such as shigellosis and amebiasis, in which the causative organism can usually be identified, and diseases that are presumed noninfectious, such as Crohn's disease (also known as granulomatous colitis or regional enteritis); most of these diseases have pathological features different from those of ulcerative colitis. The differential diagnosis is discussed in more detail in Chapter 9. Although ulcerative colitis is sometimes diagnosed by exclusion, its true diagnosis is according to a definition by specific pathological criteria (see Chapter 4).

THE PRINCIPAL FEATURES OF ULCERATIVE COLITIS

Ulcerative colitis is an inflammatory disease of the mucosa of the large intestine, with extension to the submucosa only in severe cases. It typically involves the rectum down to the anal margin, extending in continuity for a variable distance proximally in the colon. In its maximal extent it can involve the entire colon. In some patients the rectum is apparently spared, but there are always histological abnormalities in the rectum. A mild inflammation of the ileum ("backwash ileitis") sometimes occurs in patients with ulcerative colitis involving the whole colon, but otherwise the disease is confined to the large intestine.

A Homogeneous Entity

A group of British workers have applied the mathematical technique of cluster analysis to over 100 clinical, pathological, and radiological parameters in a series of patients with inflammatory bowel disease (ulcerative colitis and Crohn's disease). They found that the patients with ulcerative colitis formed a single cluster, making it a high probability that a single disease process is involved. On the other hand, their patients with Crohn's disease fell into six different clusters, suggesting that that disease may be a more heterogeneous entity (1).

ULCERATIVE PROCTITIS

The term "ulcerative proctitis" is used to describe patients in whom the sigmoidoscopic changes of ulcerative colitis are limited to the lower 10 cm or so of the rectum. Alternative names are *hemorrhagic proctitis* and *idiopathic proctitis*. The histological features in the involved part of the rectum are the same as in ulcerative colitis, but the prognosis is much more benign than with more extensive colitis. There is no reason to believe that ulcerative proctitis is any different from ulcerative colitis, except for its more limited extent. In a recent study, similar immunological abnormalities were found in colonoscopic biopsy specimens from the inflamed rectum and from apparently uninvolved proximal parts of the colon in patients with ulcerative proctitis (2).

THE PHYSICIAN AND THE PATIENT WITH ULCERATIVE COLITIS

Modern therapeutic medicine (including surgery) is probably overestimated in Western society in respect of its contribution to prolonged survival, especially compared to the benefits of good nutrition, hygiene, and preventive medicine. However, for the patient with ulcerative colitis of more than the mildest variety, the intervention of the physician can have a great influence on survival and on symptoms and general health. Severe ulcerative colitis is, by natural history, frequently a fatal disease, and it can be fatal even in the hands of the best physicians and surgeons. Corticosteroids, intravenous blood and fluid replacement, and surgical resection of the colon can, each of them, be lifesaving in specific situations; yet corticosteroids and surgery can also endanger life and must be employed correctly and skillfully.

Ulcerative colitis is a disease that rarely remits completely. The person who has once suffered from an attack of ulcerative colitis, however mild, must be regarded henceforth as having the disease and is at risk of having further attacks and eventually of colonic carcinoma developing as a complication of the colitis. He or she can benefit greatly from being seen at least twice a year by a physician with experience in treating the inflammatory bowel diseases, so that unsuspected disease activity can be suppressed. The patient should get in touch with this physician whenever symptoms suggest an impending flare-up of the disease. Anyone who has had the disease for more than seven years needs a six-monthly sigmoidoscopy, preferably with a biopsy, for the early detection of colonic carcinoma (see Chapter 15).

Persons with chronic diseases such as ulcerative colitis frequently go from physician to physician in the search for a cure, or, at least, for a cure that does not involve a permanent ileostomy. Provided that reputable and experienced physicians are consulted, this need not be deprecated; and it is to be encouraged if a specialist rather than a general physician is sought. Often the sufferer is renewed in the confidence to deal with the disease by receiving fresh advice, even though this may be of little or no additional benefit with regard to the progress of the disease. The patient's trust in the primary physician may be restored by a concurring second opinion.

The danger in this situation is that the patient may leave the care of one interested physician and no longer receive ongoing medical care, either through a failure to find another physician or through the failure or inability of the new consultant to provide continuing care, perhaps because his practice is located in another city. The patient whose specialist physician is in another city should also have a reliable family practitioner who can be consulted in an emergency and who is familiar with the program of the specialist physician and is able and willing to be in touch with the specialist.

2

EPIDEMIOLOGY

DIAGNOSTIC DIFFICULTIES

The problem with defining accurately the incidence of any disease in a community is the impossibility of being certain that the existence of the disease has been sought in every member of that community. Even if concern is restricted to the incidence of symptomatic disease, persons with symptoms may not present themselves to a physician or the diagnosis may not be correctly made when they do. Diagnostic criteria are not well defined with many diseases, especially in disorders such as ulcerative colitis in which there is no identifiable infectious agent and in which death or surgery is not an inevitable outcome. On the other hand, the practicing physician only needs an approximate notion of the incidence of diseases in order to estimate the likelihood that a given patient will have a particular disease.

The present-day physician can diagnose typical cases of ulcerative colitis with a fair degree of accuracy, especially if he is prepared to perform sigmoidoscopy on patients with suggestive symptoms and to take biopsy specimens through the sigmoidoscope when the appearances are suspicious but perhaps not diagnostic. The problem in the past, and to some extent today, has been to differentiate ulcerative colitis from the formerly much more common infectious diseases of the colon, such as shigellosis and amebiasis. In many parts of the world today, these infectious diseases are so prevalent that limited medical services frequently presume the diagnosis of an infectious dysentery.

Ulcerative colitis as a chronic nonbacterial, nonprotozoal disease has been recognized since the end of the 19th century, following the emergence of modern bacteriology and the elucidation of Koch's postulates, which enabled the bacterial and protozoal dysenteries to be identified. The lax use of terms such as "mucous colitis" and "spastic colitis" to describe the irritable colon syndrome, which is certainly not a form of inflammatory colitis, has at times confused the lay public; but informed physicians have always been aware of the differences between functional and inflammatory bowel diseases, even if they have not always succeeded in making an accurate diagnosis in the individual patient.

On the other hand, there has been a good deal of confusion in medical circles between ulcerative colitis and Crohn's disease of the colon. Burrill B. Crohn described terminal ileitis in 1932 (3); and its counterpart in the colon, granulomatous colitis, was described in 1934 (4). Yet there was a delay of 20 to 30 years before there was widespread awareness that Crohn's disease could affect the colon and the rectum, as well as the small intestine (5).

A further difficulty has been the question of whether or not to include cases of ulcerative or hemorrhagic proctitis under the heading of ulcerative colitis. In ulcerative proctitis the histology of the mucosa is similar to that in ulcerative colitis, and there is no reason to consider that it is more than a milder and less extensive form of ulcerative colitis. There is no demarcation between ulcerative colitis and ulcerative proctitis. From an epidemiological point of view, there is greater difficulty in the designation of the mildest forms of proctitis, in which the inflammation as seen by histology is often not sufficient to be diagnostic for ulcerative colitis; thus, figures for the incidence of ulcerative colitis can be greatly influenced by the cutoff point for the inclusion of patients with mild or doubtful affliction.

A STEADY INCIDENCE

Good epidemiological studies of the incidence of ulcerative colitis and Crohn's disease have been available from the United States, Great Britain, and Scandinavia from about the mid-1950s. They appear to show a steady incidence of ulcerative colitis which can be contrasted with a rising incidence of Crohn's disease by two- to threefold between 1958 and 1973 reported in studies from Nottingham, England (6), and Malmö, Sweden (7).

INCIDENCE AND PREVALENCE

The annual incidence of a disease in a community is the proportion of that community which is newly afflicted with that disease in a single year. One has to distinguish between the incidence of diagnosed disease and that of undiagnosed disease, and this depends on the proportion of affected patients who are diagnosed in life. If the vast majority of sufferers are eventually correctly diagnosed (and if a negligible number of patients are incorrectly given the diagnosis), then there will be little difference between the incidence of actual disease and the incidence of diagnosed disease, provided there is no significant change in the rate at which affected persons are positively diagnosed.

The annual incidence of diagnosed ulcerative colitis in the United States and Northern Europe is approximately 5 to 10 per 100,000 population. For Crohn's disease the incidence is probably between 3 and 5 per 100,000, so that ulcerative colitis is still more common than Crohn's disease, by a ratio of about 1.5 to 2:1.

The prevalence of a disease means the number of affected persons as a proportion of a total population, and it matters a great deal how diligently the disease is diagnosed. The person who has once suffered from ulcerative colitis remains liable to relapse and is rarely without some histological evidence of the disease. The assumption is made that ulcerative colitis is a chronic disorder that does not remit completely from the biological point of view, and patients who have had a total colectomy are included by this definition. Therefore, the prevalence of the diagnosed disease is the multiple of the annual incidence and the number of years of mean survival from the time of diagnosis. The latter figure is, of course, dependent on the mean age of diagnosis and on the mortality of the disease. Taking all persons with ulcerative colitis, the life expectancy is not greatly shortened nowadays (see Chapter 20). With a mean age of onset of 25 to 30 and a mean survival of 20 to 30 years, the prevalence of ulcerative colitis by this calculation should be 100 to 300 per 100,000 population. The measured estimates of the prevalence are closer to 100 per 100,000 population, or 1 in 1,000.

PERSONAL FACTORS

Age

Ulcerative colitis can occur at any age. One of the authors has taken care of a patient in whom the disease started at the age of 6 weeks (the case is well documented). Onset in very early childhood is unusual, but onset in the teens and early 20s is very common; roughly 50% of patients have their first symptoms of disease between the ages of 10 and 30. There is a small secondary peak in incidence at the age of 60 (Figure 2–1), patients with onset at a later age have a more benign course of the disease although a lesser ability to withstand its effects.

Sex

Acheson in England in the early 1960s reported the female to male ratio for ulcerative colitis at 1.3:1 (8), but many subsequent series have not shown this sex

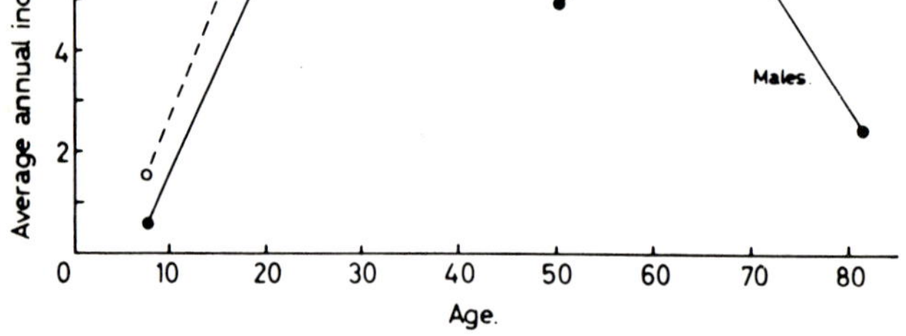

FIGURE 2–1
Annual incidence of ulcerative colitis at different ages in males and females in the Oxford area of England in the 1950s, as determined by Evans and Acheson (8). (Reproduced by permission of the authors and the Editor of *Gut*.)

difference. In particular, it has not been apparent in any United States series. If there is a female excess, it is so small as to be of no help in evaluating the probabilities of the diagnosis in a given patient.

Race and Geography

Ulcerative colitis has been seen most in the countries with the most developed medical diagnostic services, and its differentiation from the infectious bowel diseases so widespread in poorer countries requires facilities that are generally not available in those areas. As advanced medical services reach some populations that previously did not have such well-established services, the incidence of ulcerative colitis has appeared to increase from a low level, although the puzzle remains that the rise in the incidence of the disease has been slower than the presumed improvement in diagnostic capability. Examples of such populations have been those of Japan, of the American blacks, and of Asians from the Indian subcontinent living in Western Europe and North America. In Japan and among black Americans and American Indians, the incidence of ulcerative colitis appears to be considerably less than among white populations. In one racial group, the Jews, the incidence appears to be two to four times that of non-Jewish white neighbors, although the Jews in Israel do not seem to have as much colitis as the Jews in Europe and North America (9).

Social Status

The higher incidence of ulcerative colitis in the richer countries suggests that some social factors may influence the occurrence of this disease. Series originating from referral centers are of relatively little value in this respect because of the considerations that influence a patient to seek treatment at a referral center. One Danish study has shown a higher incidence of ulcerative colitis among higher socioeconomic groups (10), but most other studies have failed to reveal any social or economic factors that affect the incidence of ulcerative colitis.

HEREDITARY FACTORS

Strict Mendelian inheritance of ulcerative colitis has not been shown to occur, but there is a definite increased familial incidence of the disease. Of course, the diagnosis of ulcerative colitis in one member of a family will increase the index of suspicion in other members of the family, so that it is difficult to give a figure to the likelihood of familial occurrence. Between 10 and 20% of sufferers do have an affected relative. There seems no increased tendency for spouses and other nonconsanguineous relatives to acquire the disease.

Genetic Relationship to Crohn's Disease

The relationship between ulcerative colitis and Crohn's disease becomes interesting in this context because it is not uncommon for families to have several members with inflammatory bowel disease, some of whom have ulcerative colitis and some of whom have Crohn's disease. A person with ulcerative colitis is more likely to have a relative with Crohn's disease than is a person without bowel disease, although he is more likely to have a relative with ulcerative colitis than one with Crohn's disease.

The Likelihood of Genetic Transmission

It would be difficult to tell a prospective parent who has the disease what the chances are that a child will be afflicted. They are certainly less than 10%. Ulcerative colitis is not sufficiently prevalent for there to be significant numbers of couples in which both partners have the disease; by analogy with other diseases for which there is a hereditary tendency, the probability that a child of such a marriage will be affected may be around 10 to 20%, but probably no more than this.

3

ETIOLOGY

A DISEASE OF UNKNOWN ETIOLOGY

The cause of ulcerative colitis remains in question. There are a number of clues, but at the moment they are no more than pointers. If further work places these clues on a more solid basis, then one may anticipate the finding that ulcerative colitis results from a genetically determined immunological reaction to a viral agent. Such a viral agent has not yet been identified, although there has been one report of a candidate particle (11).

GENETIC INFLUENCES

The familial occurrence of ulcerative colitis was mentioned in the previous chapter. The inherited tendency to ulcerative colitis only infrequently leads to the actual development of the disease, so that the genes involved must have a low penetrance. In one series from Birmingham, England, there was an increased incidence of the HL-A 7 histocompatibility gene among a group of patients with ulcerative colitis compared to controls; and there were other differences in the histocompatibility antigen profile between the colitics and the controls (12). However, there was no antigen that was invariably present among the patients with ulcerative colitis. These results are probably just a reflection of a multifactorial genetic tendency to acquire the disease. One cannot state from these data whether the disease develops entirely because of the fortuitous association of a number of genes or whether there is an environmental as well as a genetic element.

AN INFECTIOUS AGENT?

There is one indirect piece of evidence of an environmental factor in ulcerative colitis. Strickland and his colleagues have demonstrated an increased incidence of lymphocytotoxic antibodies in patients with ulcerative colitis, compared to matched controls, and there was also an increased incidence of this antibody in both the blood relatives and the spouses of the colitic patients (13). As far as the authors are aware, this is the only piece of epidemiological evidence that is suggestive of a transmissible infectious agent in ulcerative colitis.

Cave and co-workers in London appear to have produced lesions similar to those of human ulcerative colitis in rabbits into which homogenized and filtered colonic tissue from human patients with ulcerative colitis was injected (14). Tissue from patients without inflammatory bowel disease did not produce such lesions. Tissue taken from the rabbits which developed the lesions then induced similar lesions when injected into another group of rabbits. The transmissible factor could pass a 100-nm filter. It took many months for the lesions to develop in the rabbits, and the assumption drawn is that if an infectious agent is the cause of these phenomena, it must be small (less than 100 nm) and slow in its induction of evident disease. A slow virus is the suggestion. The same group of workers have performed similar experiments with tissue from patients with Crohn's disease and have demonstrated similar transmissibility, although the morphology of the lesions produced was slightly different (15). As with many other features of ulcerative colitis and Crohn's disease, there may well be a common etiology for these two conditions.

Gitnick and Rosen in Los Angeles (11) have now reported finding a 120-nm viral-like particle in rabbit ileal tissue cultures inoculated with tissue from patients with ulcerative colitis. The particle was cytopathic in tissue culture and had physical and chemical characteristics similar to those of a particle they isolated from tissues of patients with Crohn's disease, although the Crohn's disease particle was smaller in size.

However, no known microorganism has yet been shown to be present in abnormal amounts in patients with ulcerative colitis; nor has any organism been shown to be able to transmit the disease in human beings.

AN IMMUNOLOGICAL DISORDER

A variety of immunological abnormalities have been demonstrated in patients with ulcerative colitis. These could be primary phenomena, occurring as a consequence of a certain inherited genotype; or they could be a response to an environmental abnormality. A possible explanation is that they are the result of an inherited type of immune reaction to a particular set of environmental circumstances. The colon is an organ containing vast numbers of many bacterial species; so one might expect that colonic bacteria are in some way involved in the etiology of the disease. The bacteria (or other types of microorganism) may be the primary cause of the disease in susceptible people; or they may be responsible for the development of a lesion that other factors have initiated.

An example of an immune phenomenon noted among patients with ulcerative colitis is the increased incidence of an antibody to *Escherichia coli* strain 0:14 (16). This is a humoral antibody and may just be a marker of the presence of damaged colonic mucosa. One learns more about the etiology of the disease from the work of Jewell and Macllennan, who have demonstrated circulating immune complexes in the serum of about one-third of patients with ulcerative colitis (17). It may be that immune complexes are deposited in the colonic mucosa and thereby cause the disease, but the origin of the immune complexes remains a mystery. The extracolonic manifestations of ulcerative colitis (arthritis, uveitis, etc.) resemble those seen in the autoimmune group of diseases, such as systemic lupus erythematosus, in which there are circulating immune complexes in high titer. Some cell-mediated immune phenomena have been shown to be altered in ulcerative colitis. In particular, lymphocytes cytotoxic for the colonic epithelial cell have been demonstrated (18), but it is difficult to conceive of this as primary rather than secondary, because this feature does not outlast for more than a few days the removal of the colon at total colectomy.

The most that one can say at the moment is that among patients with ulcerative colitis there are some abnormal features in certain immunological tests, particularly tests involving the human colonic epithelium and *E. coli* strain 0:14. From an etiological point of view, the favorable clinical response of the disease to immunosuppressive agents such as corticosteroids and azathioprine supports the opinion that some immunological mechanisms are involved, at least in part, in the development of ulcerative colitis.

RELATIONSHIPS TO CROHN'S DISEASE

Crohn's disease and ulcerative colitis have many features in common. They both usually present with diarrhea, rectal bleeding, abdominal pain, fever, or weight loss, and they are both ulcerating inflammatory diseases of the intestine, both of unknown etiology. The diagnostic differentiation of the two conditions is often difficult, and occasionally a colectomy specimen shows features of both diseases. They have identical extracolonic manifestations (joint, eye, liver, and skin disorders); and there are families in which some members of the family have ulcerative colitis, whereas others have Crohn's disease. Some physicians use the term inflammatory bowel disease to refer to the two disorders, implying their close similarity.

Ulcerative colitis is a more acute inflammatory disease than Crohn's disease. Immunohistochemical studies of the lamina propria indicate that in ulcerative colitis IgE-containing cells are found, indicating a reaginic immune process (19). In Crohn's disease, IgE cells are not found, but there are more IgA-containing cells than in ulcerative colitis (20). However, immunological studies have in general revealed more similarities than differences between ulcerative colitis and Crohn's disease. The incidence of atopic disorders is higher than normal in both conditions, and immune complexes have been found in the sera of patients with both disorders.

One can speculate about the relationship between the two forms of inflammatory bowel disease. Perhaps they represent different forms of immune response to the same environmental antigen, taking an analogy in the differing reactions of different persons to the hepatitis B antigen. One cannot help feeling that there is some etiological relevance in the fact that ulcerative colitis does not spread proximally from the large intestine with its luxuriant bacterial flora into the small intestine with its relative sterility, whereas Crohn's disease has a predilection for the ileocecal valve, which is the boundary between the differing bacterial environments of small and large bowel.

RELATIONSHIPS TO OTHER DISEASES

Ulcerative colitis (and Crohn's disease) is frequently associated with inflammatory lesions of the joints, the eyes, and the skin which are similar to those found in the rheumatic group of diseases, such as rheumatoid arthritis, systemic lupus erythematosus, and the recently identified entity called the mixed connective tissue disease. In the latter diseases, there are circulating antibodies to immunoglobulins and to nucleic acids, and the similarity of the lesions to many of the lesions of ulcerative colitis supports the idea of an immunological mechanism for these extracolonic lesions. The recent demonstration by immunofluorescence of an antibody to a C-type virus in the kidneys of patients with systemic lupus erythematosus (21) leads one to wonder whether there may not be a viral etiology for all the rheumatoid and the inflammatory bowel diseases, with the lesions of these diseases resulting from the immunological response to the virus.

MILK AND ULCERATIVE COLITIS

Truelove stimulated some excitement in the early 1960s when he reported that a proportion of his patients with ulcerative colitis remitted when placed on a milk-free diet (22). Neither his nor any other laboratory has been able to identify an immunological form of allergy to milk in patients with ulcerative colitis. Milk allergy seen in young children does not seem to be related to ulcerative colitis. The only clue in this story is that Truelove himself has reported that patients with ulcerative colitis who also had hypolactasia of the small intestinal mucosa (a genetically determined state that is widespread in the world and cannot be considered to be genuinely pathological) had more severe attacks of the disease than patients who had normal intestinal lactase, although there was no increased incidence of hypolactasia in a large group of patients with ulcerative colitis of all grades of severity (23).

ULCERATIVE COLITIS AS A PSYCHOSOMATIC DISORDER

That ulcerative colitis has a psychosomatic basis has been and remains a popular concept; yet a psychological influence on the occurrence of ulcerative colitis remains unproved by controlled studies. Lay people and uninformed physicians sometimes confuse ulcerative colitis and the irritable colon syndrome. In the latter, clear associations between emotional factors and this symptomatic disorder have been shown in a number of well-controlled studies. With regard to ulcerative colitis, the feeling of many physicians is that the persons who acquire the disease are often introspective and compulsive and that attacks of the disease are apt to follow major crises in their lives. One study, however, could not detect any difference from control patients in the incidence of preceding life crises (24). On the other hand, a report of depressed T-lymphocyte function in bereaved patients (25) may allow a cellular explanation for crisis-related relapse of an immunological disorder such as ulcerative colitis.

One is left with three alternative possibilities: 1) that the association between psychological factors and ulcerative colitis is apparent rather than real, with the more compulsive and dependent patients demanding more of the physician's time, being prepared to accept nothing less than "normal" pain-free bowel function, and taking themselves to see more than one physician, which often involves the referral centers which tend to be the sources of writings on the subject; 2) that the association with psychological disturbances is a real one but the methods available for psychological measurement are too crude or the workers in the field have not been sufficiently skillful to demonstrate the relationship in a scientifically acceptable manner; 3) that there is an element of truth in both of these hypotheses, with the association being less than is apparent, but real though not great enough to have yet been proved.

One possible theory is that the incidence of ulcerative colitis is not related to psychological factors but that the emotionally upset person has an increased intestinal motor activity (this has been shown in the irritable colon syndrome) which can interfere with the healing of the bowel in an attack of the disease, making clinical attacks of the disease more common and more severe than in a more emotionally stable person. The apparent psychological disturbances may be entirely secondary to the symptoms as appreciated by the affected person. The occurrence of this disease in older children and in adolescents may inevitably lead to the sorts of personality traits that physicians perceive in these patients and to the overprotectiveness observed in their parents.

4

PATHOLOGY

ANATOMICAL DISTRIBUTION

Ulcerative colitis is a disease of the large intestine. A mild and limited degree of inflammation is sometimes seen in the terminal ileum in patients with ulcerative colitis involving the whole colon ("backwash ileitis"), and there are a number of systemic extracolonic lesions that can occur (see Chapter 8); but backwash ileitis and most of the extracolonic manifestations regress when the colon is removed. However, the primary disease is confined to the colon, with the appendix sometimes being involved and sometimes not.

In patients with ulcerative colitis, the mucosa of the colon is inflamed continuously in a single segment of disease (unlike the "skip" lesions that can occur in Crohn's disease). In the majority of cases, the involved segment extends proximally from the anal margin, terminating at some point in the colon where the inflamed colon changes to a normal appearance over a length of 3 cm or so. It is quite common for the disease to involve the whole colon, in which case the inflammation will terminate abruptly at the ileocecal valve (except perhaps for a mild degree of backwash ileal inflammation).

The disease is frequently microscopically more extensive than is seen macroscopically. The mucosa proximal to the limit of macroscopic involvement often shows a mild inflammatory infiltrate. There are patients in whom the rectum appears to be spared, judging from macroscopic examination, but the rectal mucosa always shows evidence of the disease when it is examined under the microscope. Thus, one can say that rectal involvement is an essential feature of the disease. A few patients with ulcerative colitis do have *relative* rectal sparing; it can be seen secondarily in patients taking corticosteroid enemas or suppositories. However, the finding of rectal sparing should make one alert for the alternative diagnosis of Crohn's disease.

MACROSCOPIC APPEARANCES

The macroscopic appearances of ulcerative colitis depend, of course, on the severity of the colitis.

In mild cases, there is a fine granularity of the mucosa, with hyperemia. This progresses to mucosal edema, and then ulcerations can develop. These can be of any size, from small petechial ulcerations to deeper linear ulcers. The ulcers can be isolated, or they can be continuous and linear, in which case there can be islands of inflamed but intact mucosa between them (Figure 4–1). In severe cases, large areas of the colon can be denuded of their mucosa (Figure 4–2). Ulcerated areas have a surface of granulation tissue. Although the affected segment of the colon is a continuous one, there can be variation in the degree of activity, so that a patchy appearance can result. The intact mucosa can become thickened as a result of edema.

In patients who have chronic disease, the alternating processes of ulceration with granulation tissue formation followed by re-epithelialization and recovery can lead to the development of polypoid processes on the mucosa. These are not neoplastic, and they are termed *pseudopolyps,* although they are genuine polyps by an anatomical definition. There may be isolated polyps, or the mucosa may be carpeted with them. They can form bridges, with a single polyp being attached at two points on the surface of the mucosa. A case of intestinal obstruction due to a large pseudopolyp has recently been described in a patient with ulcerative colitis (26). Polyps occur less frequently in the rectum than elsewhere in the colon.

Following an episode of active inflammation, the disease often enters a quiescent phase. The mucosa is no longer entirely normal, either microscopically or macroscopically. The macroscopic abnormality is best appreciated on endoscopic examination when the mucosa frequently has lost its glistening appearance and the submucosal network of blood vessels is no longer visible. Hyperemia has remitted.

In a pathological specimen these features can be difficult to appreciate. The surface is usually not as smooth as that of a normal colon; alternatively, it can be flat and atrophic.

Long-standing disease gives rise to hyperplasia of the muscularis mucosae, and this, sometimes accompanied by postinflammatory fibrosis, causes shortening of the colon. The haustrations are lost, and the organ appears like a straight tube. This fibromuscular hyperplasia can be localized and gives rise to strictures which can be short or long. These then need to be distinguished from malignant

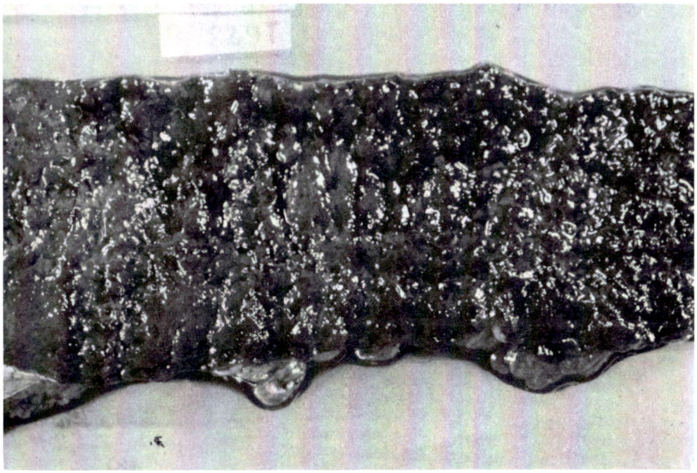

FIGURE 4–1
Severely ulcerated colonic mucosa in ulcerative colitis (pathological specimen).

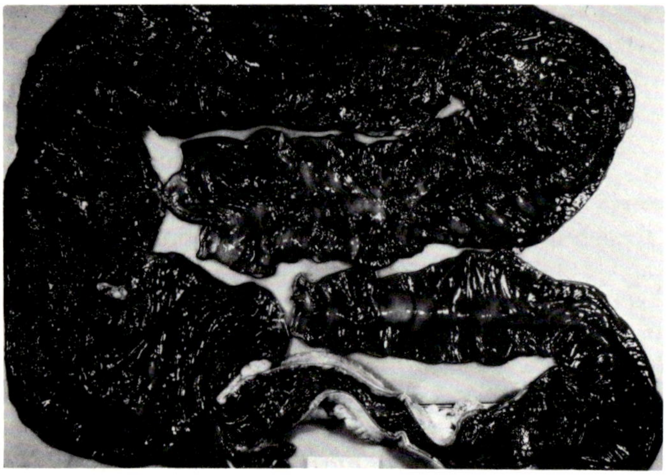

FIGURE 4–2
Toxic dilatation of the colon complicating ulcerative colitis (pathological specimen). The cecum is in the *upper center* of the field and the rectum in the *lower center*. The dilatation is most marked in the transverse colon (lying in the *left* and *upper* parts of the field) and can also be seen in the sigmoid colon *(lower right)*. The descending colon *(bottom)* is narrow.

strictures, which can also complicate ulcerative colitis. The benign strictures are smoother in their form, and, of course, microscopic examination of tissue from the stricture reveals their benign nature.

Although ulcerative colitis is primarily a mucosal disease, the inflammation in a severe case can involve the submucosa and the serosa; and the serosal surface can then be seen to be inflamed with a fibrinous exudate on it. Perforation can occur, and the sites of perforation will then be apparent on examination of the serosal aspect of the colon. Abscess cavities can form in relation to the perforations.

In toxic dilatation of the colon, which is a particularly acute form of ulcerative colitis, the diameter of the lumen of the colon is greatly increased. This process occurs preferentially in the transverse colon and the cecum (see Chapter 7), but any part of the colon, except the rectum, can be affected. The colon is blown up like a balloon. The reason for this is not clear, but it may be due to local hypokalemia and paralysis of the outer smooth muscle. The bowel wall becomes very thin and congested with dilated blood vessels, besides showing the features of severe colitis (Figure 4–2). The thin bowel wall is easily torn by handling at surgery (and on examination of the removed specimen), and the combination of a high intraluminal pressure and a fragile bowel wall commonly leads to perforation and peritonitis.

MICROSCOPIC APPEARANCES

The normal colonic mucosa consists of an epithelium with fairly close and regularly spaced crypts. The surface layer of this epithelium contains columnar cells and many mucus-containing goblet cells. Between the crypts are the mesothelial cells of the lamina propria—mainly plasma cells, lymphocytes, and macrophages. Beneath the lamina propria is the muscularis mucosae, and the crypts dip down as far as the muscularis (Figure 4–3).

In ulcerative colitis and also in other forms of colitis, the inflammation commences in the lamina propria, where increased numbers of inflammatory cells expand the lamina propria. In this layer are also seen dilated capillaries. In ulcerative colitis, these inflammatory cells include plasma cells, lymphocytes, and monocytes in most cases, eosinophils in many cases, and polymorphonuclear leukocytes in acute and subacute cases. The hyperemia and the inflammation cause the lamina propria to become slightly edematous. The inflammatory cells destroy the epithelium, so that in the severest forms of colitis (in ulcerative colitis and in other forms of colitis) the epithelium is lost and there is only granulation tissue in place of epithelium and lamina propria. At that end stage, it is difficult to diagnose the nature of the colitis. Thus, the mildest forms and the most severe forms of ulcerative colitis are the most difficult to differentiate from other diseases. Diagnostic biopsy specimens should not be taken from denuded epithelium; nor should they be taken from very mildly affected areas. In practice, however, mucosa showing typical features of ulcerative colitis can usually be sampled at endoscopy or a postsurgical or postmortem examination.

In ulcerative colitis, the presence of eosinophils is a useful diagnostic pointer. Polymorphs are also indicators of ulcerative colitis (if an infectious dysentery can be excluded). The polymorphs are typically found in the lumen of

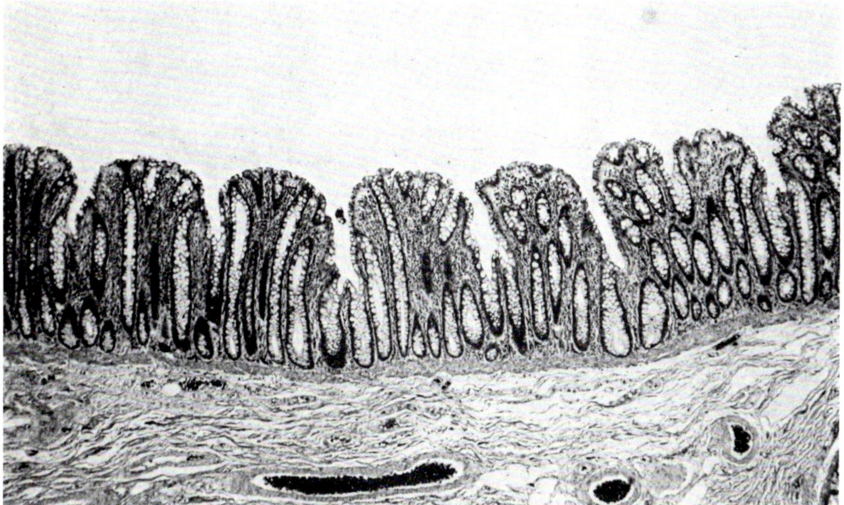

FIGURE 4–3
Histological section of normal colonic mucosa.

the base of the crypts, which they distend, causing the classical crypt abscesses (Figure 4–4). These collections of polymorphs then destroy the surrounding crypt epithelium, and the crypt abscesses become collections of polymorphs without epithelial cells at places that were previously the bases of the crypts. The inflammation proceeds to damage the crypts before there is damage to the surface epithelium. At this stage, pus cells are seen on the surface of the epithelium. The crypts make attempts at regeneration and give rise to two more typical microscopic lesions of ulcerative colitis, namely, goblet cell depletion and crypt distortion (Figure 4–5).

In the crypts, the goblet cells become replaced by columnar cells, and when present, this lesion is almost diagnostic of ulcerative colitis, being rarely seen in other forms of colitis. It is seen in the mucosa in about 50% of colons removed surgically for ulcerative colitis (27). The cause of this lesion has not been fully explained. It is probable that goblet cells develop from precursors that look like (and may be) columnar cells and that the columnar cells that replace the goblet cells in the crypts in ulcerative colitis are really immature goblet cells. It is known that in ulcerative colitis the turnover rate of the epithelium is increased (28).

As the crypts are damaged and regenerate, they become distorted. The number of crypts is diminished, with a wider lamina propria resulting. The crypts become of uneven depth, and they often branch. Once there has been a mild-to-moderate attack of ulcerative colitis, there is usually some residual abnormality of crypt morphology, even though the goblet cell complement

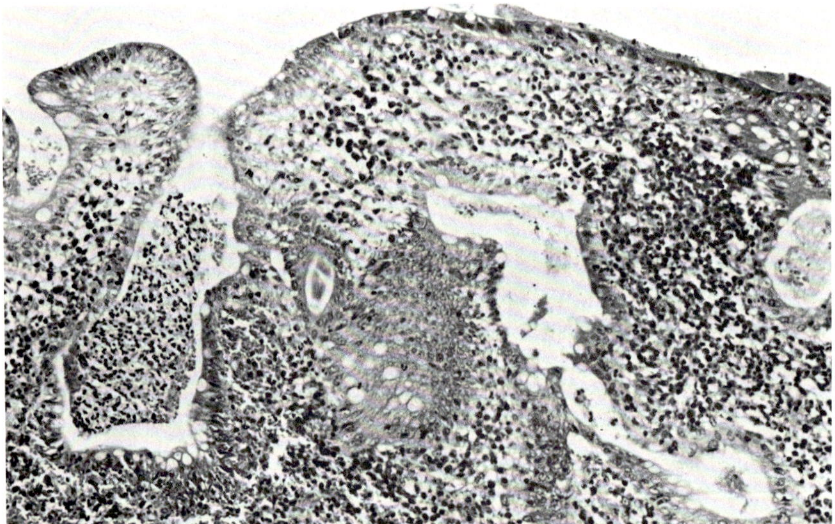

FIGURE 4–4
Histological section of colonic mucosa in acute ulcerative colitis, showing acute inflammation of the lamina propria and a crypt abscess *(center left)*.

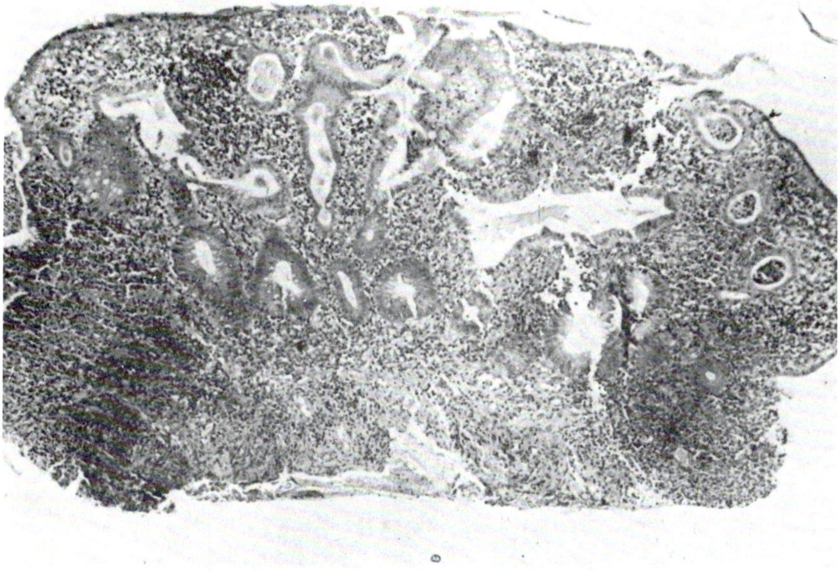

FIGURE 4–5
Lower-power view of histological section of Figure 4–4. Three crypt abscesses are seen on the *right* of the field. Crypts in which the goblet cells are replaced by columnar cells are seen in the *center* of the field.

frequently returns to normal. Thus, in inactive ulcerative colitis, in patients whose disease is giving them no symptoms and may not have done so for many years, the crypts are generally somewhat more widely spaced than normal, and they are a little distorted and often do not reach down to the muscularis mucosae.

Another change that is occasionally seen in localized areas of mucosa is a gross hypertrophy of the mucus-secreting crypts, with distension of the crypts by goblet cells containing large amounts of mucus.

In long-standing ulcerative colitis, Paneth cell metaplasia can develop among the epithelial cells at the bases of the crypts.

In quiescent ulcerative colitis, the lymphoid aggregates that are normally found in the lamina propria become larger and more prominent, and they can displace the muscularis mucosae.

In acute and severe cases of ulcerative colitis, the inflammation is not limited by the muscularis mucosae. The inflammatory cells can invade all the muscle layers to involve the serosa, and perforation with abscess formation or peritonitis can result.

The hypertrophy of the muscularis mucosae which is common in ulcerative colitis can be seen in microscopic sections (biopsies must be deep enough for this to be apparent).

EPITHELIAL DYSPLASIA

Dysplastic changes can be seen in the crypt and sometimes in the surface epithelium in ulcerative colitis. These are usually seen in the columnar cells that have replaced the goblet cells, but they can be found in goblet cells. The normal basal polarity of the cells is lost, so that the nuclei are hyperchromatic and are seen more towards the lumen of the crypt rather than basally along the basement membrane (Figure 4–6). The mucus globule in the goblet cell is often seen on the basal rather than the luminal aspect of the cell, and disorganized goblet cell hyperplasia is sometimes seen. The nuclei can assume atypical forms (nuclear polymorphism), and entire cells can acquire abnormal shapes.

These dysplastic changes can be found in regenerating mucosa following acute inflammation. In these circumstances they have no special significance,

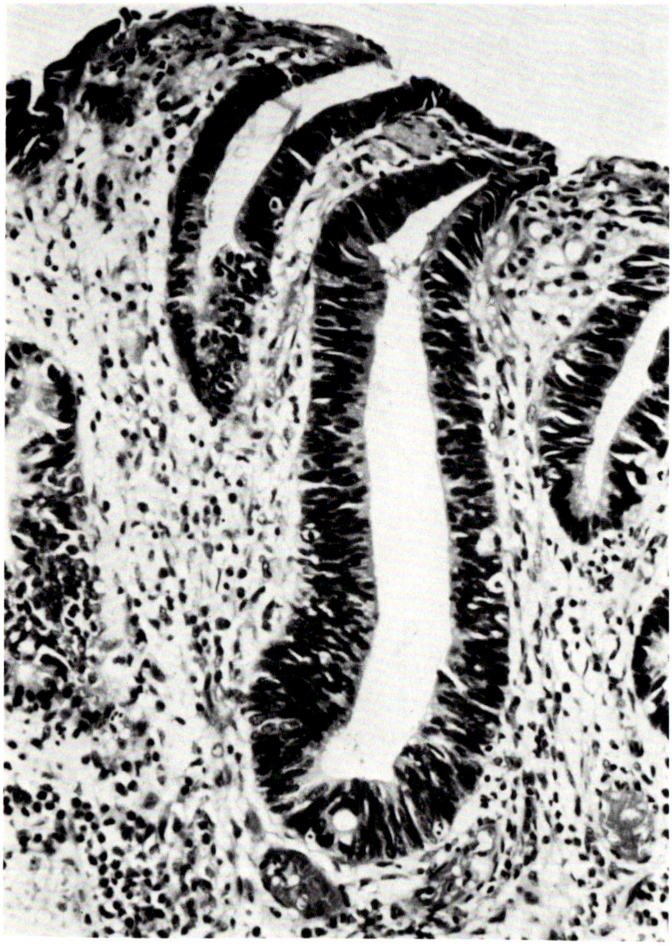

FIGURE 4–6
Epithelial dysplasia in the colonic mucosal crypts in ulcerative colitis. Note the loss of the normal basal polarity of the nuclear chromatin in the epithelial cells.

apart from indicating the degree of severity of the colitis. When found in mucosa that is not inflamed, they are now considered by many pathologists to signify a premalignant state. Severe dysplasia in rectal or colonoscopic biopsy specimens is now being taken in many medical centers, including the authors', as an indication for a prophylactic proctocolectomy in a patient with ulcerative colitis of more than seven years' duration (see Chapter 15).

CARCINOMA COMPLICATING ULCERATIVE COLITIS

The colonic mucosa in ulcerative colitis has a premalignant potential, and patients with long-standing disease are at special risk of carcinoma of the colon. The tumors that develop have the same spectrum of pathological appearances as carcinoma of the colon is noncolitics, but the incidence of particular features is weighted. The distribution tends to be more proximal in colitic patients than in noncolitics, with fewer of the tumors accessible to sigmoidoscopy, unfortunately. Sessile forms are also commoner, so that intramucosal and even deep spread has frequently occurred before the lesions can be detected in the lumen.

Although the majority of polyps in ulcerative colitis are pseudopolyps, adenomatous polyps also occur more often than in noncolitic patients; and they have the same forms and the same low but measurable premalignant potential. The presence of an adenomatous polyp probably indicates that the colitic mucosa has more of a premalignant tendency than would otherwise be the case. Pseudopolyps themselves are not premalignant and do not develop into adenomatous polyps. However, if dysplastic premalignant changes are present in the mucosa they are especially likely to be apparent in pseudopolyps. Also, the presence of pseudopolyps implies that the colitis is not of the mildest degree and therefore there is a greater risk of carcinoma than with very mild forms of the disease.

ANAL LESIONS

In ulcerative colitis there can be anal fissures that can develop into fistulous tracks to the skin, to the vagina, and occasionally to the bladder. Fistulization is by no means as common in ulcerative colitis as in Crohn's disease; and the inflammation in ulcerative colitis includes polymorphs of more acute inflammation.

PERIPHERAL COMPLICATIONS OF ULCERATIVE COLITIS

The pathology of the peripheral complications of ulcerative colitis is discussed in Chapter 8, together with a description of each complication.

DIFFERENTIAL DIAGNOSIS (29)

Ulcerative colitis must be distinguished pathologically from a number of other inflammatory diseases of the colon that are described below. The clinical differential diagnosis of ulcerative colitis is considered in Chapter 9.

Acute Dysentery

In acute dysentery caused by the *Shigella* species of gram-negative rods, the colon is diffusely involved in a superficial mucosal inflammatory process. The process is not limited to the distal part of the colon. Microscopically, the acute inflammation is very similar to that of ulcerative colitis, and in the majority of cases the two cannot be distinguished solely on their biopsy features. There are acute inflammatory lesions, with polymorphs predominating, together with crypt abscesses. However, the lesion heals completely, so that the regenerative features of the crypts found in ulcerative colitis are absent in dysentery and goblet cell depletion is unusual. Microbiological cultures are required to make the diagnosis of bacillary dysentery.

Amebiasis

Amebic dysentery also involves the whole colon, but the inflammation is a little less acute than with bacillary dysentery. There is mucosal inflammation, and crypt abscesses form. There is a greater tendency than in ulcerative colitis for only the bases of the crypts to be involved in the crypt abscesses, so that the well-known flask-shaped ulcers develop, narrow superficially, and wider more deeply. On the other hand, ulceration between the crypts is more common than in ulcerative colitis. Microscopically, both in the mucosa and in adherent mucus, the vegetative forms of *Entamoeba histolytica* should be sought and can often, but not always, be found. They sometimes contain ingested red blood cells; in the mucosa they can be seen surrounded by a zone of necrosis. In chronic amebiasis, mucosal inflammatory excrescences can develop which resemble carcinomas on barium enema X-ray examination; but these contain the parasite and are known as amebomas.

Other Protozoal Infections

Balantidium coli produces a lesion that resembles amebiasis but is more predominantly right-sided in the colon. The protozoa can be seen in histological sections.

Schmistosoma mansoni and *Schistosoma japonicum* can infest the colon, mainly the rectum and distal colon. The inflammation is more chronic and granulomatous than that of ulcerative colitis. There is an intense granulomatous reaction surrounding the eggs of the parasite in the mucosa.

Other Infections

Lymphogranuloma venereum, caused by *Bedsonia* virus, can inflame the rectum. The histology is less acute than in ulcerative colitis.

The colon can be involved in tuberculous infections. The cecum is the commonest site. The lesions resemble those of Crohn's disease rather than those of ulcerative colitis. Acid-fast bacilli are found in relation to giant cells.

Histoplasmosis and *candidiasis* are fungal diseases that can cause inflammatory lesions in the colon and rectum. They are being seen more often with the increasing use of immunosuppressant and other antitumor drugs. The inflammation they cause is of a more chronic type than that of ulcerative colitis.

Crohn's Disease

The differentiation of Crohn's disease from ulcerative colitis is one of the commonest diagnostic problems in clinical gastroenterology. In Crohn's disease, the large bowel can be spared entirely. More often there is cecal and right-sided involvement, but any part or all of the colon, including the rectum, can be affected. Skip lesions, with apparently normal mucosa intervening, are a common finding.

The inflammatory reaction in Crohn's disease generally lacks polymorphs (although a few can be seen) and is mainly composed of round cells (lymphocytes and monocytes), plasma cells, and macrophages. Epithelioid granulomas, frequently containing giant cells, often can be seen in the submucosa and sometimes in the muscle and serosal layer, but the granuloma is not an essential component in the lesion of Crohn's disease. Even though the lamina propria is the prime site of the inflammation, causing mucosal edema, the inflammatory process tends to progress to deeper layers, involving the serosa, with postinflammatory fibrosis. The epithelium is less affected than in ulcerative colitis. Ulcers do form, though these are often deep fissures involving the muscular layers. The finding of superficial ulcers does not exclude Crohn's disease, and in fact the presence of small aphthoid ulcers is a recently recognized feature of Crohn's disease; these are characterized by microabscesses deep in the lamina propria which are larger, fewer, and more discrete than the crypt abscesses of ulcerative colitis. In severe cases of Crohn's disease, there is the same epithelial destruction as in ulcerative colitis. However, disordered regeneration of crypts is less marked than in ulcerative colitis, and goblet cell depletion is an unusual finding, except immediately adjacent to fissures. There is lymphatic dilatation and a certain degree of vascular dilatation in all layers. In the submucosa, lymphoid aggregates are seen. The edema of the bowel surface together with the linear fissuring ulcers gives rise to the well-known cobblestone appearance on macroscopic examination of the mucosa.

The full-thickness inflammation causes edematous and fibrotic thickening and narrowing of the bowel, and pericolic abscesses form from fissuring ulcers, which also give rise to fistulous tracks. These fistulas are lined with granulation tissue and often contain giant-cell granulomas. Fistulas can lead to the perianal or abdominal skin, to other parts of the bowel (e.g., gastrocolic and enterocolic fistulas), and to the vagina and to the urinary tract. However, the mucosal surface in Crohn's disease of the colon can at times appear very similar to that in ulcerative colitis. Pseudopolyps can be found in Crohn's disease, toxic dilatation can occur, and carcinoma can complicate the disease; however, these features are less frequent than in ulcerative colitis.

Ischemic Colitis

Ischemic colitis is a form of colitis that is usually localized to one segment of the colon, most often in the ascending colon or at the splenic flexure but sometimes in the rectum. It is a reaction to ischemia of the mucosa caused by arterial disease, or sometimes in association with use of the contraceptive pill. The superficial epithelium and the more superficial parts of the crypts become necrotic, and there is considerable vascular congestion and edema of the lamina propria. Occasionally a fibrin thrombus can be seen in a mucosal or submucosal capillary. The entire mucosa can necrose, but otherwise healing occurs, leaving a distorted crypt pattern but without gross goblet cell depletion. Fibrosis in the lamina propria can ensue, with stricture formation.

Membranous Colitis

A membranous colitis, which is also known as pseudomembranous colitis, is apt to occur following the use of broad-spectrum antibiotics. Recently it has been described especially after the use of lincomycin or clindamycin. Following antibiotic therapy, some patients have massive staphylococcal infection, this being known as staphylococcal enterocolitis, but the lesion is the same as in membranous colitis without staphylococcal infection. It can also occur without prior antibiotic use, particularly if there has been hypotension or hypoxia associated with cardiopulmonary disease or major surgery. The lesion was thought to be different from that of ischemic colitis, but it probably is an ischemic form of colitis caused by fibrin-plugging of mucosal capillaries. The small intestine, as well as the colon, may be involved, and the colonic lesion is more often diffuse than in ischemic colitis.

Macroscopically, the mucosa is hyperemic and edematous but not granular. White plaques form which can then necrose, leaving a mucosa with ulcerated areas. Microscopically, the lesion is often patchy in relation to focuses of fibrinoid necrosis. There is intense mucosal and submucosal vascular congestion, with dilatation of capillaries and some edema. The superficial epithelium becomes replaced by a loosely adherent membrane of fibrin, mucus, and pus cells. The deeper crypts hypertrophy and become distended with mucus, although this is not an invariable feature. The condition can progress to a full-thickness inflammation and to perforation and death; but more often it remains mucosal and heals completely.

Radiation Colitis

Acute congestive and inflammatory changes are seen in the rectum in the days following irradiation to the uterine cervix, but these soon heal. More often confused with ulcerative colitis are rectal lesions coming on months or years after the radiation therapy. The submucosal blood vessels become hyalinized, and there is dilatation of the mucosal capillaries. A mild inflammatory infiltrate is present in the lamina propria, and ulceration can occur, though crypt abscesses are not seen. The crypts can become atrophic and sometimes distorted, but there is no goblet cell depletion.

Solitary Rectal Ulcer Syndrome

In the solitary rectal ulcer syndrome, found particularly in young adults (especially women), and possibly caused by spasm of the pubococcygeus muscle, a granular ulcerated area is seen in the rectum, usually on the anterior wall, about 8 to 10 cm from the anal margin. Biopsy distinguishes this from ulcerative colitis. The histological features are the same as those of prolapsed colonic mucosa. The surface epithelium can become ulcerated, and there is a mild inflammatory infiltrate. A pathognomonic feature is strands of smooth muscle in the lamina propria between the crypts. The muscularis mucosae is thickened. In the deeper layers, glandular tissue may be seen which has arisen as a result of reparative processes; and it gives rise to the appearance known as "colitis cystica profunda," which is part of the solitary ulcer syndrome.

Cathartic Colon

The colonic mucosal appearances that result from prolonged use of the senna and cascara groups of purgatives should not occasion the erroneous diagnosis of ulcerative colitis. There is sometimes an excess of chronic inflammatory cells in the lamina propria, and there may be mild edema of the lamina propria, but the epithelium and the crypts are entirely normal. A diagnostic finding is the presence of brown pigment in macrophages in the mucosa, which is known as melanosis coli, and can often be appreciated on sigmoidoscopy. The muscularis mucosae may become thickened.

Irritable Colon Syndrome

In theory, there should never be any difficulty in the histological differentiation of ulcerative colitis and the irritable colon syndrome. In the irritable colon syndrome, the bowel is entirely normal, and this should be apparent on rectal biopsy. In practice, it may be tricky to decide whether a very mild inflammatory infiltrate is normal, indicating the irritable colon syndrome, or is sufficiently abnormal to be labeled as ulcerative colitis. At times, one cannot give a certain opinion; however, ulcerative colitis of such a mild degree would have a good prognosis in any event.

There is a pitfall in the diagnosis of ulcerative colitis following preparation for sigmoidoscopy with a Fleet enema or with topical bisacodyl. These agents can cause detachment of the surface epithelium (although the crypts are unaffected), and they can also induce a mild polymorph infiltrate into the mucosa, so that a normal mucosa can erroneously be thought of as showing ulcerative colitis.

II

The Clinical Presentation

5

SYMPTOMS

The astute clinician can often suspect ulcerative colitis on the basis of the patient's history alone, even before sigmoidoscopy or a radiological study of the colon has been performed. However, many other disorders can mimic ulcerative colitis in their clinical presentation, including the extremely common conditions of infectious diarrhea and hemorrhoids (see Chapter 9). The five most common symptoms of ulcerative colitis are rectal bleeding, diarrhea, abdominal pain, weight loss, and fever, in that order of frequency. The severity of all of these symptoms correlates with the extent of the colitis in the colon and with the severity of the inflammation. In mild cases there are fewer symptoms. When the disease is in remission, there are often no symptoms whatsoever. It also occasionally happens that persons with active disease are free of symptoms, or the symptoms cause so little disability that they are ignored; however, it is unusual for the person with moderately active ulcerative colitis not to have one or more of these symptoms, and it is virtually impossible for anyone to have severe ulcerative colitis without any symptoms.

RECTAL BLEEDING

The most frequent symptom of ulcerative colitis, and often the first symptom, is the passage of blood from the rectum. This symptom may be discounted by the patient as being due to hemorrhoids. Alternatively, it may provoke alarm and suggest to the patient the possibility of carcinoma of the colon. An important clue to the diagnosis of ulcerative colitis is the passage of mucus with the blood, with or without diarrhea.

In the distal forms of ulcerative colitis (such as ulcerative proctitis), blood and mucus accumulate in the rectum, to be passed when sufficient irritation induces the patient to pass a stool. The blood and mucus are often passed without stool of any kind, or they are passed only when a scybalous stool moves through the rectum. Some patients come to expect a certain amount of rectal bleeding to be a persistent feature of their disease, though the total elimination of rectal bleeding is an important therapeutic goal in the management of ulcerative colitis.

In the more severe cases, when the disease has spread proximally, the amount of rectal bleeding may be considerable. The degree of bleeding is roughly proportional to the extent of the disease (unlike the situation in Crohn's disease, in which heavy bleeding can occur from a single deep fissured ulcer even if the disease is of limited extent). In the acutely ill patient with transmural involvement with ulcerative colitis, torrential bleeding may occur, leading to hypotension and shock, with the hazard of acute renal failure.

Occult Bleeding

Occult rectal bleeding, detected only by chemical testing of the stool by guaiac or Hemoccult, can also lead to the diagnosis of ulcerative colitis. Patients with other suggestive symptoms of ulcerative colitis, such as abdominal pain or diarrhea, or with an iron-deficiency anemia, should be tested for occult bleeding. In many patients occult bleeding is discovered during the course of a medical examination for another illness or as part of a medical checkup. It is doubtful whether testing for occult bleeding is of any value in the management of the patient with diagnosed ulcerative colitis. A certain amount of microscopic bleeding which does not cause anemia is probably inevitable in many patients.

Pathophysiology

Microscopic bleeding from each of the myriads of tiny ulcers combines to produce the symptom of macroscopic bleeding in patients with mild and moderate ulcerative colitis. In severe colitis, macroscopic bleeding can occur from individual large ulcers and from denuded areas of mucosa. Larger vessels may be eroded as the ulceration increases in severity. Heavy bleeding in acute colitis may be due to lack of constriction of the vasa vasorum.

Some theories relate the bleeding in ulcerative colitis to local ischemia of the colonic mucosa as a result of vasospasm or of localized thrombosis of the small vessels in the mucosa. The similarities between ischemic colitis and ulcerative colitis are often quoted to support these theories. However, phenoxybenzamine (Dibenzyline), a powerful vasodilator, has been unsuccessful as therapy to arrest colonic bleeding in ulterative colitis. Localized thrombosis has been demonstrated on rectal biopsy in patients with ulcerative colitis. Excessive fibrinolytic activity has been reported on rectal biopsy of patients with ulcerative colitis, and this has been proposed as a mechanism for the bleeding (30). Treatment with topical epsilon-aminocaproic acid has been advocated, but there are no convincing reports of the successful use of that form of therapy.

DIARRHEA

The most disabling symptom of ulcerative colitis is urgent diarrhea. Many patients with ulcerative colitis have diarrhea without urgency, which can be a tolerable situation if therapy cannot bring it totally under control. Diarrhea is defined as the passage of loose or watery but not necessarily frequent stools. However, the increase in stool frequency that often accompanies the diarrhea of ulcerative colitis can be more troublesome than the diarrhea itself. In the most acute forms of ulcerative colitis, the patient can have diarrhea more than twenty times in 24 hours. The diarrhea is apt to occur particularly after meals and as the patient wakes up in the morning. It may persist through the night, robbing patients of their sleep and aggravating the debilitating effects of the disease. The functional diarrhea of the irritable colon syndrome hardly ever wakes the patient in the middle of the night, and this is a useful differential feature for the physician.

Urgency of stool can exist with or without diarrhea. Patients may experience such urgency that they lose bowel control and soil their clothes. Such embarrassing accidents lead to a loss of self-esteem and have an adverse effect on the patient's emotional state.

Diarrhea is not an inevitable symptom in ulcerative colitis. Patients with ulcerative proctitis may not suffer at all from diarrhea. Patients in whom the colitis is in remission are often free of diarrhea.

Pus in the Stools

Some patients with active ulcerative colitis complain of the passage of purulent material in their stools. This usually accompanies diarrhea or bleeding. However, the pus may leak through the anus in between bowel movements. A heavy flow of pus suggests a perianal fistula or an abscess draining from the perianal area or via the rectum or sigmoid colon.

Mucus in the Stools

The passage of clear-colored mucus is frequent in ulcerative colitis. In fact, the complaint of passing pus may, on inspection of the material, turn out to be simply excessive colonic mucus. In ulcerative colitis the passage of mucus in the stools generally accompanies diarrhea or bleeding, whereas in the irritable colon syndrome (in which the passage of mucus is also common) the mucus is more likely to accompany formed stools; this distinction is not invariable.

Pathophysiology

Physiologically, diarrhea is due to an increase in the water weight of the stool due to decreased water absorption. The small bowel presents around 1,500 ml of liquid contents to the colon each day, but the daily stool volume is normally only about 200 ml. It is easy to appreciate how a small decrease in colonic salt and water absorption will result in increased amounts of fecal water. In ulcerative colitis the damaged mucosa is unable to absorb salt and water. It is the right side of the colon where the majority of the water is absorbed; hence, in extensive ulcerative colitis there is more severe diarrhea than when the disease is limited to the left side of the colon. Water absorption may be impaired when mucosal inflammation damages the epithelium; in severe cases the epithelium may be absent in large areas of the colon.

When the colonic mucosa is severely inflamed, the contiguous mucosal cell layer is no longer intact and there is leakage of serum and extracellular fluid into the colon (31). Also, the inflammatory reaction in the colonic mucosa stimulates, probably via a cholinergic mechanism, an increase in mucus secretion by the colonic goblet cells (32).

Chronic ulcerative colitis causes shortening of the large intestine as a result of muscular hyperplasia, thereby diminishing its capacity to retain fecal fluid for sufficient time for achievement of the salt and water re-absorption of which the mucosa is still capable. There is fecal hurry through the shortened colon.

Urgency of stool in ulcerative colitis can be explained by two mechanisms that interact with each other. These are a reflex resulting from inflammatory irritation in the rectum and the effects of exaggerated and more frequent mass peristaltic movements of the colon propelling the fecal contents into the rectum.

Malabsorption with steatorrhea has not been recorded in ulcerative colitis. If these features are detected, an alternative diagnosis should be considered. Most commonly, the disease proves to be Crohn's disease involving the small intestine.

Constipation

Constipation is an unusual symptom of left-sided ulcerative colitis. The stool impacts in the uninvolved colon proximal to the affected area. The patient may continue to experience diarrhea, but physical examination and X-ray examination will demonstrate the retained stool in the right side of the colon.

ABDOMINAL PAIN

In the acutely ill patient with ulcerative colitis, abdominal pain may be intense, especially if the inflammation is involving the serosal layers of the colon. Serosal inflammation in the severely ill patient causes a constant aching discomfort, often associated with hypoactive bowel sounds and some degree of rebound tenderness. This may be a prelude to toxic dilatation of the colon. If the pain is distinctly localized, it may indicate a pericolic abscess.

Otherwise, abdominal pain is usually not a prominent feature of ulcerative colitis. To be sure, cramping is a daily occurrence in some patients with ulcerative colitis, but usually it is relieved by defecation and is not a chronic discomfort. In contrast, the pain in Crohn's colitis tends to be a more prominent and frequent feature. The pain of ulcerative colitis is especially apt to occur 30 to 90 minutes after a meal, and this may lead the patient or an inexperienced physician to ascribe the symptom to a gastric or duodenal ulcer.

Pathophysiology

Colonic pain is caused in some cases by stretching of the smooth muscle and in other cases by serosal inflammation, though these mechanisms can be operative simultaneously. Stretching of the colon is responsible for intense cramping and urgency prior to defecation, and it results from mass peristalsis with distension and contraction of various areas of the colon. Active or previously active ulcerative colitis results, in many cases, in disturbance of the normally well-coordinated colonic motility. This is the same mechanism that is present in the painful irritable colon syndrome, but it is apt to be more intense and more intolerable in ulcerative colitis. Muscular strictures seen in the colon in ulcerative colitis illustrate the severity of the disordered motility.

Postprandial pain is the result of the mass peristalsis that normally follows a meal. This is elicited by a "gastrocolic reflex," which is ill understood; its mechanism may involve the action on the colon of cholecystokinin (CCK) released from the jejunal mucosa.

RECTAL PAIN

Pain in ulcerative colitis may also be experienced in the rectum. One form of rectal pain is tenesmus, a severe bearing-down pain lasting for many minutes and usually accompanied by an inability to defecate. Tenesmus must be distinguished from proctalgia fugax, a condition not unduly associated with ulcerative colitis which is due to spasm of the levator ani sling muscles surrounding the rectum.

The mechanism of tenesmus is unclear and may represent strong contractions of an empty but irritated rectum or else excessive contractions of the internal anal sphincter.

SYSTEMIC SYMPTOMS

The systemic symptoms of ulcerative colitis can be divided into three categories: those resulting from the inflammatory process in the colon; those secondary to losses of blood and chemicals through the inflamed mucosa (or to the failure of normal colonic absorption); and those that appear to be due to some form of immune hypersensitivity reaction. In the first category are fever, weakness, and weight loss. The second category also includes weight loss and weakness; in children, there may also be growth retardation. Symptoms due to extracolonic hypersensitivity reactions include those due to inflammation of the eyes, the joints, and the skin (erythema nodosum, pyoderma gangrenosum); this group of symptoms will be discussed in Chapter 8. Fever is a sign rather than a symptom and will be discussed in Chapter 6.

Weight Loss

There are three factors that cause weight loss in ulcerative colitis: diminished intake, excessive loss of nutrients, and increased catabolism.

Diminished Intake

The chronic inflammatory process may result in anorexia from depressive effects (of unknown mechanism) on the hypothalamic appetite center. There is also often a voluntary reduction in intake if the patient experiences postprandial abdominal pain and diarrhea. To avoid these symptoms, the patient limits the amount of food he eats and loses weight for this reason. Some patients experience nausea with ulcerative colitis, and they too limit their intake. Vomiting is unusual in ulcerative colitis, although it does occur from time to time.

Therapeutic dietary restriction is another cause of weight loss. Acutely ill patients are frequently placed on light diets or fluid diets or even on totally intravenous alimentation (see Chapter 13).

Excessive Loss of Nutrients

Blood and protein losses through the inflamed colonic mucosa of ulcerative colitis patients deplete the body of amino acids and also of iron.

Hypercatabolism

In severe ulcerative colitis, an intense catabolic process occurs, even if the patient is taking in adequate amounts of calories and amino acids. Fever aggravates this catabolic state. In addition, liver disease associated with ulcerative colitis may result in diminished protein synthesis (see Chapter 8).

Corticosteroids may add to the catabolic process by augmenting gluconeogenesis. This may be apparent before one can detect beneficial effects from suppression of the inflammation. As discussed in Chapter 13, the anti-inflammatory action of corticosteroids is often suboptimal in the severely malnourished patient.

Weakness

During active ulcerative colitis, patients often are unable to perform their activities normally because of profound weakness and easy fatigability. Usually several causes combine to produce weakness, including anemia, weight loss, fever, and dehydration and loss of sodium and potassium. Emotional problems may add to the fatigue, leading, for instance, to depression, with attendant loss of self-esteem and a feeling of hopelessness.

Growth Retardation

One of the most devastating long-term effects of ulcerative colitis in children is the retardation of growth. This complication appears to be secondary to the presence of active inflammation, since growth resumes upon remission of the disease or total colectomy. The combination of active inflammation and chronic debility seems to suppress both the pituitary release of growth hormone and a target response to exogenous hormone. Loss of protein through the inflamed colon is an important factor leading to retardation of growth.

Growth retardation is a better term than growth failure, since bone age lags lies behind chronological age and epiphyseal fusion may occur long after the onset of puberty. The proper timing of surgery in children with continued active ulcerative colitis remains one of the most difficult decisions for the physician, since physical and psychosocial factors must be carefully weighed. This subject will be discussed further in Chapter 18.

6

PHYSICAL SIGNS

The diagnosis of ulcerative colitis is based on the clinical history, on objective findings derived from sigmoidoscopy (or colonoscopy), often combined with a biopsy, and on radiological studies (which will be discussed in later chapters). Most physical signs in ulcerative colitis represent complications of the disease. Physical signs of some noncolonic complications of ulcerative colitis can be attributed in a general way to a "hypersensitivity" reaction. As discussed in Chapter 3, the mechanisms for these inflammatory responses far from the site of origin are poorly understood, although they do seem to be directly related in some way to the activity of the disease. Other signs are secondary to poor nutrition, including anemia and hypoproteinemia.

GENERAL APPEARANCE

Often the astute physician can detect the activity and severity of the ulcerative colitis by his initial impression of the patient. The pale, wan, anxious patient suggests significant disease, particularly if he was healthy when the physician saw him previously. Anemia is common in ulcerative colitis (see Chapter 8) and can usually be detected from the appearance of the nail beds and the mucosae.

The loss of muscle mass in fulminant ulcerative colitis is striking and often may occur within a short time after the onset of the disease, reflecting profound catabolism. Chronic diarrhea with the loss of protein from the gastrointestinal tract may also be responsible for the loss of muscle mass.

There are associations between certain skin conditions (e.g., erythema nodosum, pyoderma gangrenosum) and ulcerative colitis. The skin should be examined carefully for evidence of these and of possible drug rashes. The cutaneous complications of ulcerative colitis are discussed in Chapter 8.

FEVER

The inflammatory nature of ulcerative colitis results in a pyrexia in many patients with active disease. The fever is roughly proportional to the activity of the disease. Fever is not an inevitable feature, but its presence indicates certainly that the activity of the colitis is at least in the moderate rather than the mild category. A high temperature (exceeding 39°C) can be due to severe colitis without a specific complication, such as perforation, peritonitis, septicemia, or abscess formation. Resolution of a fever most often reflects recovery from the acute attack, but this can be a false sign since overwhelming disease can suppress the body's pyrogenic responses; and also corticosteroids by themselves depress the body temperature without necessarily curing the underlying condition, e.g., when there is perforation of the colon.

Fever can also be a symptom of one or more of the extracolonic complications of ulcerative colitis, such as arthritis or pericholangitis, or of an intercurrent complication such as a urinary tract infection or venous thrombosis. Fever can also be a manifestation of a drug reaction, particularly a reaction to sulfasalazine.

THE EXTREMITIES

Clubbing can occur in long-standing, moderately severe ulcerative colitis that involves the ascending colon. It can also occur when cirrhosis complicates ulcerative colitis. The presence of clubbing does not seem to be a guide to the development of colonic carcinoma. The actual mechanism of clubbing is unknown. Hypertrophic osteoarthropathy has also been reported in ulcerative colitis (33), though it is unusual.

Since various forms of arthritis can complicate ulcerative colitis, the joints should be examined carefully. Details of abnormalities in the joints are discussed in Chapter 8.

THE MOUTH

Dehydration in acute ulcerative colitis may be appreciated by seeing a dry, furred tongue.

Aphthous stomatitis is relatively common among the population at large, but it occurs more commonly and often rather severely in patients with ulcerative colitis. The ulcers may be larger than are usually seen, and they may be extremely painful, often contributing to the depressed nutrition of the patient. The oral ulceration may be on the mucous membranes of the mouth or on the palate.

THE ABDOMINAL EXAMINATION

In most patients with ulcerative colitis, the examination of the abdomen is unremarkable. Tenderness over the sigmoid is often present. However, the sigmoid can also be tender in patients with the irritable colon syndrome and in normal individuals.

In the severely ill patient with fulminant ulcerative colitis, the abdominal examination becomes extremely important. This part of the examination should be performed several times each day. The onset of tenderness over the colon, particularly with rebound, in an acutely ill patient with fever and extreme diarrhea often signals the onset of "pericolitis," suggesting that the inflammatory process is extending beyond the mucosa and rendering the colon vulnerable to perforation. Attention to bowel sounds can be most helpful to the examiner, since a decrease is suggestive of the development of a toxic megacolon. Percussion of the colon also is valuable, particularly when performed repeatedly. A tympanitic colon with bowel sounds absent should be considered as an indication of a toxic dilatation until this is excluded by evidence of abdominal x-ray films. Sometimes the edge of a dilated transverse can be palpated—it feels like a child's balloon just beneath the abdominal wall.

The finding of a mass within the abdomen raises the suspicion of a tumor or an abscess. If the mass is in the right lower quadrant, Crohn's disease should be suspected as an alternative diagnosis. Confusion may arise from the presence of hard stools in a constipated colon; the stool may impact in a normal ascending or transverse colon proximal to left-sided ulcerative colitis.

Other findings in the abdomen are unusual. Hepatomegaly is rare, even in the presence of pericholangitis, unless cirrhosis is present. If there is portal hypertension complicating the cirrhosis, the spleen may be palpable.

THE RECTAL EXAMINATION

The perianal area should be examined carefully, first visually and then digitally. A rectal examination should always precede sigmoidoscopy, since disease in the anal canal may cause pain or insertion of the sigmoidoscope.

Anal fistulas usually can be viewed without difficulty on inspection of the anal area. Some anal fissures can be seen by the examiner if he spreads apart the patient's buttocks with his hands and looks closely at the anal area, whereas other fissures can only be visualized endoscopically.

Digital examination should be performed carefully if an anal fissure is suspected, since pain will be produced. In the case of a fissure, the little finger rather than the index finger in the anal canal may cause less discomfort to the patient and may yield sufficient information. Gentle pressure against the fissure will produce discomfort, while pressure against other areas will not. Although most fissures are usually located posteriorly, fissures associated with inflammatory bowel disease may be in any location; so an atypical fissure should raise the suspicion of inflammatory bowel disease. Perianal abscesses can also be detected by the digital rectal examination.

Bidigital examination is often overlooked; yet this may be extremely helpful in delineating a perianal abscess or the track of a fistula. The index finger is placed in the anal canal, and the perianal tissue is palpated between the thumb and forefinger.

Some clinicians feel that the degree of inflammation of the rectal mucosa can be assessed on digital palpation, but this is questionable since the involvement is usually quite superficial. Only in situations of chronic disease with marked coarse granularity or in fulminant ulcerative colitis with wide rectal furrows can a sufficient degree of differentiation be present to be appreciated by the palpating finger. Polyps (which are usually pseudopolyps) can often be felt on rectal examination, and it should not be forgotten that carcinoma complicating ulcerative colitis can, in up to 25% of cases, be detected by a diligent rectal examination.

The presence of blood on the finger at a digital examination is an important physical sign. Testing of the stool for occult blood was discussed in Chapter 5.

OTHER ASPECTS OF THE PHYSICAL EXAMINATION

The extracolonic complications of ulcerative colitis (discussed in Chapter 8) can give rise to signs in the eyes and elsewhere, for example, in the legs (erythema nodosum, venous thrombosis). Since ulcerative colitis, even in the absence of systemic complications, frequently has general systemic effects, and since the modes of therapy, both medical and surgical, have profound systemic effects of their own, it is essential for the physican to perform a complete physical examination on a patient with ulcerative colitis, not only when he is being seen for the first time but also at the onset of a flare-up of the disease, or at least every six months during remission.

Vaginal and Pelvic Examination

There is a temptation to omit the vaginal and pelvic part of the physical examination, but this would be an error in a woman suffering from a disease that involves the rectum and perineum. However, it should be satisfactory for the physician treating the colitis to rely on recent findings reported firsthand by a reputable gynecologist.

7 LOCAL COMPLICATIONS

The complications of ulcerative colitis may involve only the colon, or there may be extracolonic complications, or a patient may have both local and systemic complications. Mild ulcerative colitis has a low incidence of complications, but as the disease becomes more severe the likelihood of complications increases.

The local complications may be classified as those associated with fulminant ulcerative colitis, those associated with chronic colitis, and those that are perianal complications.

FULMINANT ULCERATIVE COLITIS

Fulminant ulcerative colitis may arise *de novo* in a previously healthy individual, or it may occur as the culmination of a chronic relapsing course of the disease. Criteria for assessing the severity of activity of ulcerative colitis and classifying cases as being mild, moderate, or severe are considered in Chapter 10; "fulminant" ulcerative colitis refers to the most severe forms of the "severe" category. Pathologically, in fulminant ulcerative colitis there are multiple large ulcerations becoming confluent with denudation of the submucosa and resulting in a raw, bleeding surface with only a few remnants of mucosa remaining (see Figure 4–2). The progressive loss of mucosa with an irregular colonic surface can be appreciated radiologically, on a plain abdominal film (Chapter 12). In this setting, the acutely ill, toxic patient often develops one of the following colonic complications of ulcerative colitis: hemorrhage, toxic megacolon, or perforation.

HEMORRHAGE

Rectal bleeding is one of the hallmark symptoms of ulcerative colitis; yet exsanguinating hemorrhage is exceptional, and when it occurs, there is almost always severe disease. Massive hemorrhage is a relatively uncommon complication compared to perforation and toxic megacolon. Multiple transfusions and, rarely, surgery may be required to stem the uncontrollable bleeding. Otherwise, the treatment is that of severe ulcerative colitis, as outlined in Chapter 13. The pathophysiology of colonic hemorrhage in ulcerative colitis was discussed in Chapter 5.

TOXIC MEGACOLON

The acute dilatation of the colon that can occur in fulminant ulcerative colitis remains controversial with respect to its etiology and its therapy. Although toxic megacolon may occur spontaneously in severe ulcerative colitis, it is often precipitated iatrogenically by certain drugs (see below); the physician caring for a patient with severe ulcerative colitis must remember Galen's dictum: "Primum non nocere."

Pathophysiology

In toxic dilatation of the colon there appears to be a loss of tone in the colonic muscle layers, allowing the intraluminal pressure to expand the colon beyond its normal width. This mechanism can explain the effects of opiates, anticholinergic drugs, and hypokalemia. When severe ulcerative colitis extends deep to the mucosa and submucosa, the polymorphonuclear inflammatory infiltrate in the muscular layers gives rise to edema that probably impairs the contractile ability of the circular muscle.

Most often it is the proximal two-thirds of the colon that is affected by toxic dilatation. The reason for this is unclear. The transverse colon is often the first portion to be dilated, probably because of its mesentery. The next area to become dilated is the cecum, in which the muscular layers are the least developed. The cecum can enlarge more than the transverse colon, so that measuring the cecal diameter is a means of following the patient's progress and possibly of making the diagnosis. The sigmoid musculature is the thickest in the colon, so that, despite its mesentery, it does not easily dilate. Also, if bacterial toxins are an etiological factor (as discussed below), the right side of the colon, being more static, contains larger numbers of viable bacteria than the left side of the colon; this may be the reason for the higher incidence of toxic dilatation on the right side. The ascending and transverse portions of the colon are supplied by the superior mesenteric artery, whereas the descending colon receives its blood from the inferior mesenteric artery; this raises the possibility of a vascular cause for toxic megacolon. Yet, except for this simple anatomical coincidence, it is difficult to formulate an explanation for the areas of predilection of toxic dilatation solely on the basis of the vascular supply.

When the inflammation in ulcerative colitis becomes severe, toxic factors derived from the luminal bacterial contents may well be absorbed by the submucosa and the muscular layers. With the mucosa largely destroyed, the colonic wall is vulnerable to bacterial invasion; and generalized sepsis frequently accompanies toxic dilation.

Pharmacological paralysis of the colonic musculature during acute ulcerative colitis, particularly in severe colitis, is an important iatrogenic cause of toxic megacolon. During severe ulcerative colitis, the circular muscle seems to be especially sensitive to opiates and to anticholinergic drugs. Even seemingly minimal doses of atropine-like drugs can precipitate toxic megacolon in severely ill patients, particularly when administered parenterally. Frequently, a single injection has been responsible for converting an uncomplicated case of severe ulcerative colitis into one with toxic dilatation. The mechanism seems to be as a result of the inhibition of the parasympathetic nerve supply to the colon, removing an important factor in the maintenance of the muscular tonus of the bowel wall. Opiates also inhibit colonic muscle directly. The pharmacological effect of opiates in paralyzing muscular contraction becomes exaggerated in a severely ill patient with ulcerative colitis. This is unfortunate since it is exactly such a patient who needs relief of pain in a fulminant episode of ulcerative colitis.

Hypokalemia also produces paresis of smooth muscles and is a common cause of toxic megacolon. A decrease in the total body potassium may be secondary to the disease, or it may be iatrogenic. Since potassium is often lost in diarrhea of any type, a patient with ulcerative colitis may be depleted of potassium even prior to the fulminant episode. The use of corticosteroids augments the potassium loss from the bowel and may also cause renal potassium losses. The edematous, hypoalbuminemic patient may also be receiving potassium-depleting thiazide diuretics. The measured serum potassium level is an imperfect measure of the status of the much higher intracellular potassium concentrations.

Another iatrogenic precipitant of toxic dilatation is the performance of barium enema X-ray examinations during fulminant attacks of ulcerative colitis. This has been reported in some series, and the authors have experience of it happening. The etiology is probably a combination of the pressure of the barium and inadvertent introduction of air in the examination and an effect of the barium in removing more of the fragile mucosal layer. Air-contrast examinations seem particularly likely to precipitate a toxic megacolon. It is the authors' feeling that a careful barium enema examination performed by an experienced radiologist controlling the pressure of the flow of barium is less often associated with this complication that an examination done by an inexperienced resident.

Clinical Manifestations

Early symptoms of an incipient toxic megacolon are often overlooked; yet they provide a clue to initiate action before more profound abnormalities develop. The patient first notes a change in bowel habit, which appears to be an improvement, and a sudden decrease or even a cessation of defecatory urges. The physician may find a pleased patient who announces that he must be improving since the diarrhea has stopped. On examination of the abdomen, the physician notes that the bowel sounds are quiet or even absent and that early distension of the colon is present, with tympany detectable, especially over the transverse colon. Distension of the abdomen is the next physical finding; often its occurs several hours after the initial symptom. Abdominal X-ray films now begin to show the characteristic accumulation of air in the transverse colon, the cecum, or the descending colon, as described in Chapter 12.

The atonic colon in toxic dilatation is liable to be associated with atony of the small intestine. Some patients with toxic megacolon experience vomiting; this may, however, be a reflex reaction to the general toxic state of the patient.

When the colon is dilated, its entire wall is edematous with polymorphonuclear cells invading the submucosa and deeper layers. At this stage, the wall of the colon is extremely thin, resembling wet tissue paper at surgery, and is very vulnerable to spontaneous perforation. Perforation may occur at any time in the course of toxic dilatation, even when the colon appears to be deflating and responding to therapy, so that constant awareness of this potentially fatal complication must prompt frequent physical examinations and the taking of serial *upright* abdominal X-ray films. As noted below, the perforation may give only minimal symptoms and signs in the patient who is receiving corticosteroid treatment. The bowel wall in toxic dilatation may be so thin that toxic bacterial products can pass through and cause peritonitis, even without there being any macroscopic perforation.

Treatment

A team effort of physician and surgeon is extremely important at this stage in treating toxic megacolon. The surgeon should be constantly available and fully aware of the entire clinical picture, and he should have met with the patient and his family. The patient should be aware that an urgent total or subtotal colectomy and ileostomy are a distinct possibility, and a full explanation of the reasons should be given, referring to the consequences of peritonitis.

Usually, an initial period of medical therapy is undertaken in all but the most acutely ill and distended patients. The medical therapy is that for severe ulcerative colitis, as discussed in Chapter 13. If the patient fails to respond to the medical therapy or becomes worse, then there is no alternative to surgery (see Chapter 16).

Prognosis

The prognosis of the patient with toxic dilatation who successfully responds to medical therapy is still not good. The development of a toxic megacolon usually implies destruction of the colonic mucosa, so that even following recovery the colon is permanently damaged, often with pseudopolyposis. The function of the colon is impaired under these circumstances, leaving the patient chronically ill. The severe nature of the disease puts the patient in a category in which he is more vulnerable to the development of a neoplasm. Several attacks of toxic megacolon in a single patient are not uncommon, such a colon being apparently especially sensitive to this complication.

In the absence of perforation before or during the operative procedure, the chance for survival is excellent. If perforation occurs, particularly before surgery, the prognosis is guarded because of the probability of generalized peritonitis.

Prevention

In view of the dangerous nature of toxic dilatation, it is important to take measures that minimize the chance of its development. These include the vigorous and early treatment of patients with moderate or severe ulcerative colitis—even patients suspected of having ulcerative colitis in whom the diagnosis is not yet certain—and the avoidance in these patients of opiates and anticholinergic medications. Drugs to be avoided include morphine, meperidine (Demerol, pethidine); pentazocine (Talwin, Fortral); codeine (including codeine combinations, such as Tylenol and codeine preparations that are inaccurately called "Tylenol No. 1,"' "Tylenol No. 2", etc.); and dihydrocodeine (DF-118 in Great Britain). These are opiate derivatives and analogues. Also to be avoided are belladonna (often in combinations such as Bellergal); atropine and hyoscine (in combinations such as Donnatal); diphenoxylate with atropine (Lomotil); propantheline (Pro-Banthine) and other anticholinergics (e.g., Pathilon); and the new antidiarrheal agent loperamide (Imodium), which inhibits colonic peristalsis via a non-anticholinergic mechanism. The sympatomatic treatment of diarrhea and pain in severe ulcerative colitis is discussed in Chapter 13.

Avoidance of barium enema X-ray examinations during severe attacks of ulcerative colitis, or their performance only by skilled radiologists and only when they are considered essential, should also help reduce the incidence of toxic megacolon. Double-contrast barium X-ray studies should be forbidden during acute attacks of ulcerative colitis.

PERFORATION

The most life-threatening complication of ulcerative colitis is perforation of the colon. It almost always results in a generalized peritonitis because of the sudden and usually massive soilage of the peritoneal cavity. This can be followed by septicemia and shock, which may be fatal. The reason for the severity of perforation in ulcerative colitis is the tissue-paper-thin bowel wall in fulminant colitis, especially in toxic megacolon, which tends to perforate at more than one site. By contrast, the thickened colon wall in Crohn's disease more commonly produces either a localized perforation with an abscess or a fistula through various organs.

Perforation usually occurs only when there is fulminant ulcerative colitis or a toxic megacolon, although a perforation can occur in a patient with less than fulminant disease, possibly by extension of an ulcer through the layers of the bowel wall. Corticosteroids may interfere with the normal reparative process of the colonic mucosa, thus allowing deeper penetration of ulcers.

Symptoms of perforation include abdominal pain, often generalized, absence of bowel activity, and distension. Physical findings are fever, absent bowel sounds, tenderness, rebound tenderness, and sometimes a loss of hepatic dullness. Diagnostic studies reveal a marked left shift on the differential white blood cell count, often with leukocytosis, and free air on a plain upright abdominal X-ray film.

One of the major problems in the patient with ulcerative colitis and perforation is the possible masking of symptoms by corticosteroids. Thus, a patient with acute ulcerative colitis may have a perforation without experiencing fever or abdominal pain. Despite frequent admonitions regarding "silent perforation," there usually are some clinical indications, such as a change in the clinical course or, as mentioned above, the development of fever, decreased or absent bowel sounds, or an increase in the leukocyte count.

The treatment of colonic perforation in ulcerative colitis is always surgical (see Chapter 16).

The prognosis following colonic perforation is relatively poor, despite the advent of modern antibiotic regimens.

PERITONITIS WITHOUT PERFORATION

Peritonitis can complicate severe ulcerative colitis even without there being a frank perforation. The peritonitis is most likely to occur secondary to toxic dilatation. With the mucosa destroyed, bacterial products from the lumen can pass through the thinned and inflamed colon wall, causing peritonitis in the same way as if there were a perforation, though the peritonitis can be less severe than with perforation.

Peritonitis without free perforation is an absolute indication for surgery; in fact, the diagnosis of a nonperforative peritonitis can only be made at operation.

ABSCESS FORMATION

A perforation of the descending or sigmoid colon or the rectum may be walled off by the omentum, leading to a pericolic abscess, which is not quite as disastrous as a free bowel perforation. The relatively acute nature of ulcerative colitis (compared to Crohn's disease) makes pericolic abscess formation an uncommon complication of the disease. On the other hand, postoperative intra-abdominal abscesses following the surgical treatment of ulcerative colitis are very common and are one of the most serious complications of surgery (see Chapter 16). Nonperforative peritonitis, for instance in association with toxic dilatation of the colon, can also result in intra-abdominal abscess formation.

Treatment with corticosteroids is contraindicated in the presence of a pericolic abscess; their use can lead to extension of a localized abscess to a generalized peritonitis (this is a hazard even without the use of corticosteroids).

COMPLICATIONS OF CHRONIC ULCERATIVE COLITIS

Pseudopolyposis

The severely or recurrently injured colonic mucosa may respond to such injury with the development of multiple mucosal excrescences. When these are multiple and large, the term pseudopolyposis is applied. The concept that pseudopolyps are areas of relatively uninvolved colonic mucosa surrounded by denuded mucosa is probably incorrect. The development of pseudopolyps is the result of epithelialization of inflammatory excrescences. The pathology of pseudopolyps has been discussed in Chapter 4.

The patient with pseudopolyposis has often survived an episode of fulminant ulcerative colitis or toxic megacolon. When pseudopolyps are present, the entire colon is often involved with ulcerative colitis, rather than there being just left-sided disease. The implications of pseudopolyposis are the same as those of ulcerative colitis involving the entire colon. In fact, pseudopolyposis has no further significance and does not require treatment *per se.* There has been a single report of intestinal obstruction due to giant pseudopolyps (26).

The relationship between the development of carcinoma and pseudopolyposis has been studied, with no direct correlation being shown. However, since the patient with pseudopolyposis usually has extensive involvement of the colon, together with chronic and often long-standing disease, such a patient is in a relatively high-risk category for the development of a neoplasm (see below).

Stricture

A true benign fibrous stricture of the colon is most unusual in ulcerative colitis. Much more common, and typical of ulcerative colitis, are segments of the colon in which the muscularis mucosae is thickened, giving rise to benign muscular forms of stricture (see Figure 12–6). These must be distinguished from malignant carcinomatous strictures (Figure 12–8), and from edematous and fibrotic strictures that are found in Crohn's disease of the colon. Carcinoma complicating ulcerative colitis may present as a radiological or endoscopic stricture which may have typical features, such a length greater than 2 to 3 cm or an irregular contour; however, it is impossible to be sure that a short, smooth stricture, typical of benign muscular hypertrophy in ulcerative colitis, is not really a malignant stricture. An opinion that a stricture is benign can be supported by showing it to relax and open up during a barium enema X-ray examination following the intravenous administration of glucagon or Pro-Banthine. Benign strictures are usually no more than 5 cm in length. The descending colon and the sigmoid are the commonest sites.

Whenever possible, strictures should be examined colonoscopically, and biopsy specimens and brushings should be taken to make sure that there is no malignancy. Often, one is surprised how easily the colonoscope passes through a benign stricture. Even if the stricture cannot be entered with the endoscope, a brush and biopsy forceps should be passed blindly into the stricture. Once a particular stricture that is typically benign has been confirmed to be so by colonoscopy and biopsy, there seems to be no particular risk of carcinoma developing in that stricture; and follow-up colonoscopic examinations are not required for this purpose.

Multiple areas of narrowing may be present, raising concern that there may be multicentric neoplasia. However, it is not uncommon for there to be two or three segments of benign stricture; and if at colonoscopic examination only the distal stricture can be reached, there is little chance that the other strictures are malignant if there is no suggestion of that on a double-contrast barium enema X-ray examination.

Clinically, benign strictures rarely cause trouble *per se.* Very rarely, they have been known to cause colonic obstruction. An obstructing stricture is much more likely to be due to malignancy or to a misdiagnosis of Crohn's disease.

Rectal strictures, complicating long-standing ulcerative colitis, are relatively common and are also due to muscular hypertrophy. There is usually a generalized rectal narrowing, accompanied radiologically by a marked increase in the presacral, retrorectal space (see Figure 12–2). These rectal strictures are remarkably asymptomatic.

Carcinoma of the Colon

The most feared complication of chronic ulcerative colitis is the development of carcinoma of the colon. The patient in a fulminant attack of colitis is clearly in danger from his disease, and with intensive treatment many patients can be saved in that situation; but carcinoma of the colon is a complication of long-standing ulcerative colitis, and its presentation may be delayed or may be confused with activity of the colitis. For a patient with ulcerative colitis, the chance that carcinoma of the colon will develop is roughly 20 times the chance for a noncolitic—and large bowel cancer ranks in the top three malignancies in both sexes even in the absence of ulcerative colitis.

There is, in fact, a great variation in the cancer risk of patients with ulcerative colitis. There are four factors that influence greatly the liability to carcinogenesis. These are 1) the extent of the disease, 2) the length of time the colitis has been present, 3) whether or not it has been chronically active, and 4) the age of the patient at the time of diagnosis.

The incidence of carcinoma appears to be directly proportional to the extent of colonic involvement with ulcerative colitis; thus, in distal colitis affecting only the rectosigmoid there is only a small chance that cancer will develop, whereas with total involvement of the colon there is a much greater chance. The incidence of colonic carcinoma in patients with only a proctitis is so low as to be undetectably greater than that in the general population.

The duration of diagnosed disease is an important determinant of the cancer risk. Very few cancers develop when the disease has been present for less than ten years, the incidence being quite rare when the disease is of less than five years' duration. From ten years, the incidence seems to rise rather abruptly, but in a linear fashion; the longer the disease has been present beyond ten years, the greater is the liability to carcinoma.

This ten-year "period of grace" allows the patient and the physician to plan for the possibility of neoplasia and of a prophylactic colectomy. For example, a young woman can be assured that she will probably be able to complete her family during this period without having to worry about the cancer risk (however, there are other hazards of ulcerative colitis in pregnancy—see Chapter 19); or a young student can plan to complete his education. The question of prophylactic colectomy is amplified in Chapter 16.

The degree of activity of the colitis also has an important influence on the cancer risk. Patients whose clinical course has been one of continuous activity have a much higher risk than those in whom activity has been intermittent. De Dombal and co-workers (34) relate the cancer risk to "patient-years" of activity.

A young age at the time of diagnosis of ulcerative colitis was shown by Truelove (35) to be a risk factor additional to that of the duration of the disease, but it was only a marked factor when the onset was under the age of 10.

The tumors that complicate ulcerative colitis tend to be extremely vicious and are often metastatic when they are discovered. The difficulty of diagnosing carcinoma complicating ulcerative colitis lies not just in confusion between symptoms of colitis and those of colonic carcinoma. The tumors themselves tend to be flat and infiltrating, making for late diagnosis. They also tend to be more poorly differentiated than in noncolitics (see Chapter 4 for a discussion of the pathology of these tumors). Added to this, the more even distribution of the tumors throughout the colon means that they are less likely to be detected by rectal examination or by sigmoidoscopy than are colorectal carcinomas in patients not suffering from ulcerative colitis.

Two significant but unresolved issues derive from considerations of the risk of neoplasia complicating ulcerative colitis. These are the proper method of follow-up for the patients at risk (particularly those with chronic, active disease who have had colitis proximal to the splenic flexure for more than ten years), and the question of a prophylactic colectomy, that is, a colectomy mainly directed at removal of the organ at risk for carcinoma at a stage when the patient might not otherwise have needed this operation. These questions are the subject of appropriate sections of Chapters 15 and 16.

PERIANAL COMPLICATIONS

Perianal abscesses, fistulas, or fissures are probably more common in patients with ulcerative colitis than in the normal population; yet they are much less common than among patients with Crohn's disease. The actual incidence is not known, since in many series the differentiation of ulcerative colitis from Crohn's disease has not been clearly made. In ulcerative colitis most of these complications occur during periods of disease activity (which is often not the case with the perianal complications of Crohn's disease), especially when there has been a great deal of diarrhea. Perianal fissures are the commonest of these complications.

The symptoms of the perianal complications are often pain and discomfort around the anus, especially on defecation. The anal area is tender, and the patient is liable to observe a purulent discharge or bright red rectal bleeding, both of which are easily confused with symptoms of activity of the colitis.

The signs of the perianal complications are apparent on examination of the perineum, when the physician pulls the buttocks apart with gloved fingers. A fissure or a fistula may be seen or may be palpated with the examining finger. A localized tender abscess may be detected on digital examination of the perineum or of the anal canal. This should be followed by an endoscopic examination of the anal canal using a short anoscope with good illumination. Fistulas may need to be probed with a blunted sterile probe.

The treatment of these lesions is described in Chapter 14.

8

SYSTEMIC COMPLICATIONS

At times, the extracolonic complications of ulcerative colitis can be more devastating than the disease itself. Examples include blindness from uveitis and growth failure in an adolescent. These extracolonic complications can be fatal, for instance, when cirrhosis complicates ulcerative colitis. Although some of the systemic complications respond to medical therapy or to surgery, others leave irreversible residual effects or become progressive. The prognosis for any individual complication is often more a factor of the nature of the complication than of the overall progress of the colonic disease.

Many of these systemic complications appear to be part of an "autoimmune" or "hypersensitivity" disease state. The evidence for this is largely circumstantial, by analogy with other diseases (such as serum sickness and systemic lupus erythematosus) in which disordered immunity has been clearly demonstrated. Some experimental immunological evidence exists, but it is far from confirmatory. The favorable response of the systemic complications to corticosteroids may be due to the anti-inflammatory rather than the immunosuppressive effects of those drugs. Furthermore, the response to other immunosuppressive drugs, such as azathioprine, has been disappointing.

The extraintestinal complications of ulcerative colitis can be classified into three broad groups: 1) those that are apparently of a systemic "hypersensitivity" disorder—joint, eye, skin, and oral complications; 2) those that are probably secondary to portal or pelvic bacteremia or antigenemia—liver disease, thromboembolic complications; and 3) those that are secondary to the disordered physiology of the colon, i.e., to the losses of blood, fluid, electrolytes, and nutrients. Systemic complications of drugs used in ulcerative colitis should not be ignored.

By far the most common situation is for the extraintestinal complications to appear after symptoms of the colonic disease are manifest; but extracolonic lesions are sometimes observed when the physician first sees the patient, and occasionally they precede the development of colonic symptoms or even of colonic lesions. This latter situation has been observed with chronic active liver disease occurring in association with ulcerative colitis. In general, the mildest forms of ulcerative colitis are not complicated by extraintestinal manifestations, particularly if there is merely a mild proctitis. The treatment of the systemic complications of ulcerative colitis is considered in Chapter 14.

JOINT DISORDERS

There are three separate types of joint involvement in ulcerative colitis. They are distinct and are not particularly associated with one another. They are rheumatoid arthritis, sacroiliitis with or without ankylosing spondylitis, and a specific arthritis associated with inflammatory bowel disease (ulcerative colitis and Crohn's disease). There has also been a case report of hypertrophic osteoarthropathy associated with ulcerative colitis (33).

Rheumatoid Arthritis

There is an increased incidence of rheumatoid arthritis in patients with ulcerative colitis, though the two conditions usually run separate and unrelated courses in the individual patient. The rheumatoid arthritis usually is seropositive, typically involves the small joints, and responds to the usual medical measures. Occasionally, a more severe, seronegative and therapeutically unresponsive variety occurs that resembles rheumatoid arthritis in its distribution and requires corticosteroids for symptomatic relief.

Ankylosing Spondylitis, Sacroiliitis

A remarkable association has been observed between inflammatory bowel disease and ankylosing spondylitis, raising etiological speculation relating to lymphatic drainage from the colon and other anatomic-bacteriologic explanations. The usual sex predisposition of ankylosing spondylitis is 9:1 in favor of men, whereas in ulcerative colitis the ratio is about equal. Since ankylosing spondylitis is normally uncommon in women, when the physician does see it in a woman, he should seek the presence or be aware of the possible future occurrence of inflammatory bowel disease.

Ankylosing spondylitis may occur many years before or after the onset of ulcerative colitis, and it persists or may become manifest even after total colectomy. Since ankylosing spondylitis responds poorly to corticosteroids, separate therapy may be needed for the bowel and the back.

There is an important and fascinating association between histocompatibility antigens and ankylosing spondylitis. When spondylitis occurs unassociated with ulcerative colitis, the histocompatibility antigen HL-A-B27 is found in roughly 90% of patients. On the other hand, only about 50% of patients with ankylosing spondylitis who are suffering from inflammatory bowel disease have this antigen. In a further "twist" of this story, it has been found that all patients with ulcerative colitis and Crohn's disease who *do* have the HL-A-B27 antigen develop ankylosing spondylitis, and they are also more liable to have total colonic involvement with their bowel disease (36).

The spectrum of ankylosing spondylitis associated with ulcerative colitis includes some patients who have only a sacroiliitis.

The symptoms of ankylosing spondylitis are, of course, pain and stiffness in the spine. Sacroiliitis gives rise to pain in the region of the sacroiliac joints.

The signs include the loss of the normal lumbar lordosis, inability to flex or rotate the spine, and, with sacroiliitis, pain produced in the sacroiliac joints on "springing" of the anterior superior iliac spines.

The diagnosis is confirmed by radiological examination of the spine and of the sacroiliac joints (see Chapter 12 and Figure 12–10).

The Arthritis of Inflammatory Bowel Disease

Characteristically, in the specific arthritis associated with inflammatory bowel disease, the large weight-bearing joints—the hips, the knees, the ankles, the shoulders, and the elbows—are affected, whereas the small joints are the ones most often involved in rheumatoid arthritis and the back in ankylosing spondylitis. This specific arthritis is typically a *monoarthritis* or an *oligoarthritis,* affecting only one or two joints. There are some patients who also experience symptoms in the smaller joints of the hands or feet. This large-joint type of arthritis is so characteristic of inflammatory bowel disease that when arthritis of the knees occurs in a younger person, the physician should question the patient regarding any weight loss or change in bowel habit. There is a correlation between the activity of the arthritis and the activity of the bowel disease, so that they occur in concert rather than independently. On the other hand, a dissociation between the severity of the joint inflammation and of the bowel involvement may be observed. The ulcerative colitis may be quite mild; yet the disability from the joint inflammation may be severe.

An effusion may be present. The synovial fluid is not dissimilar to that in rheumatoid arthritis, although the glucose concentration in the fluid is apt to reach lower levels in rheumatoid arthritis. The synovial proliferation in the arthritis of inflammatory bowel disease is similar pathologically to that in rheumatoid arthritis, but there is no erosion of the juxta-articular bone; and this feature can be appreciated radiologically, there being no erosions and only soft-tissue swelling.

SKIN LESIONS

Two characteristic skin lesions occur in ulcerative colitis: erythema nodosum and pyoderma gangrenosum. In addition, a wide variety of nonspecific eczematoid eruptions may be present but are rarely troublesome to the patient; they tend to be confused with drug-induced eruptions, particularly those associated with sulfasalazine and the acne of high-dose steroid treatment.

Erythema Nodosum

The characteristic dull red, raised, painful nodules of erythema nodosum usually appear over the shins but can occur elsewhere on the legs. They occur as a "hypersensitivity" reaction in a wide variety of situations, including infectious processes, such as streptococcal, tuberculous, or fungal diseases, and presumably noninfectious inflammatory conditions, such as sarcoidosis. They can also complicate sulfonamide therapy (including treatment with sulfasalazine). As the inflammatory bowel diseases become more common and the infectious diseases less frequent, ulcerative colitis and Crohn's disease should be considered frequently in the investigation of a patient with erythema nodosum.

Some patients with ulcerative colitis are predisposed to recurrent attacks of erythema nodosum. Often the degree of colonic involvement with ulcerative colitis is extensive; so the presence of erythema nodosum is a sign of moderate or severe disease.

In some patients, the condition is self-limited and not disabling, whereas in other patients prompt therapy of the colitis is required (see Chapter 14). Usually, erythema nodosum clears up and does not return following total colectomy for ulcerative colitis.

Pyoderma Gangrenosum

The lesion of pyoderma gangrenosum is characteristic for inflammatory bowel disease but occasionally may be found unrelated to intestinal disease. The appearance is pathognomonic, with a painful, ulcerated area surrounded by violaceous undermined skin (Figure 8–1). Classically, the ulcers occur on the shin, especially over the medial malleolus, but they may occur anywhere on the body, often on the arms, and even on the face. The ulceration may appear unrelated to activity of the ulcerative colitis (though there is usually some activity of the colitis), and it may enlarge explosively so that a tiny area one day may become a 2 to 3 cm ulcer by the next day. It may at first appear just as a boil on the skin.

The cause of pyoderma gangrenosum is unknown. It has been speculated that it is due to an anaerobic bacterial infection, an immunologic disorder, or the breakdown of an area of erythema nodosum.

The appearance of any small ulcer or boil on the skin of a patient with ulcerative colitis is a cause for alarm because of the propensity of pyoderma gangrenosum to explosive development. Certainly, in a patient who has had pyoderma gangrenosum previously, the chance that this complication will return is sufficiently great to warrant initiating therapy promptly (see Chapter 14).

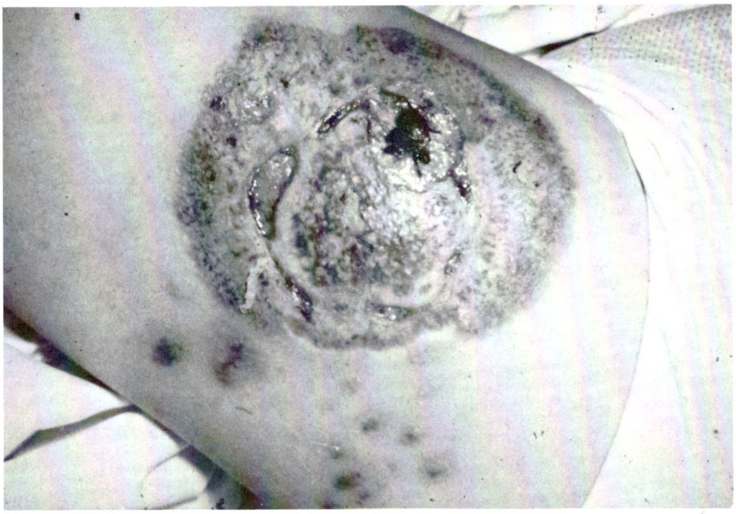

FIGURE 8–1
Advanced pyoderma gangrenosum on the thigh of a patient with ulcerative colitis.

STOMATITIS

Aphthous ulceration is one of the more common minor annoyances of many otherwise healthy people, but the type of ulceration in inflammatory bowel disease is unusual in its virulent nature; therefore, it is included among the systemic complications. The oral ulcers tend to be large, multiple, persistent, and very painful, being located anywhere in the mouth from the buccal surface to the tonsilar pillars. In some patients, mouth lesions apparently associated with ulcerative colitis may really be an oral form of Crohn's disease, but such lesions are not true aphthous ulcers; they are more cobblestoned, and their differentiation from the aphthous ulcers of inflammatory bowel disease should be possible on clinical grounds. Aphthous ulcers are found in increased frequency not only in ulcerative colitis but also in Crohn's disease and in celiac sprue.

EYE LESIONS

Three types of ocular lesion are associated with ulcerative colitis: conjunctivitis, uveitis (including iritis), and episcleritis. There is a tendency for the patient with one of these types of lesions to develop another of them. They should not be confused with the ocular complications of steroid therapy, which are glaucoma and cataract formation. Ocular lesions are much more likely to complicate chronically active than intermittently relapsing ulcerative colitis.

Conjunctivitis

Conjunctivitis, usually bilateral, is apt to occur in patients with ulcerative colitis. It is usually self-limited and causes the patient discomfort rather than disability, except when it progresses to a uveitis. The cornea and conjunctivae are red and feel gritty.

Uveitis

Uveitis is a rare yet extremely severe complication of ulcerative colitis, since blindness may result. The anterior uveal tract may be inflamed, resulting in iritis; or the posterior tract can be affected, causing retinitis.

Iritis presents as a red, painful eye, with discomfort increased in the dark, owing to pupillary dilatation. The patient's marked discomfort separates the condition from conjunctivitis. Any patient with ulcerative colitis who complains of a red, painful eye should be examined promptly by the physician and then probably by an ophthalmologist as well. Examination of the eye will reveal erythema concentrated around the iris, rather than generally or peripherally as is seen with conjunctivitis. The anterior chamber may contain condensations of inflammatory material. Cultures should be taken to exclude bacterial infection, particularly since therapy involves the use of local corticosteroids.

Posterior uveitis is much more serious and can lead to retinal destruction and blindness, particularly if the fovea is involved. Any patient with ulcerative colitis who has a sudden change in vision should be examined for posterior uveitis by a competent ophthalmologist, since prompt corticosteroid therapy may avert a disaster.

Episcleritis

Episcleritis describes inflammation of the sclera, often with localized red areas. The eye feels uncomfortable, though not as much as with uveitis. Episcleritis can be seen on examination of the eye; the patient should be asked to move his eyeball in all directions to allow a proper examination of the sclera.

HEPATOBILIARY DISORDERS

Although the liver is part of the gastrointestinal tract, its involvement in ulcerative colitis is considered here as a systemic complication. Pericholangitis is relatively common, whereas carcinoma of the bile ducts is only a recently recognized and rare complication of long-standing ulcerative colitis. When series of patients with ulcerative colitis are studied, 10 to 15% are found to have disordered liver function tests (for transaminases, alkaline phosphatase, or the sulfobromophthalein (Bromsulphalein) retention test). Needle biopsies on such patients do not always show histological abnormalities; and, likewise, patients with ulcerative colitis who for one reason or another have a liver biopsy are not always found to have abnormalities in routine liver function tests (37).

Some of the hepatobiliary disorders, such as the fatty liver, have only an incidental or a small significance for the patient; others, such as cirrhosis and sclerosing cholangitis, can cause chronic ill health and death in some cases; and biliary duct carcinoma is virtually always fatal. The prognosis of some of these disorders is improved by total colectomy, though in some cases, especially where there is an established cirrhosis, the disease progresses in spite of removal of the colon.

Fatty Liver

Among the hepatobiliary disorders, fatty liver is the commonest histological abnormality seen in patients with ulcerative colitis. It is probably indicative of the malnutrition of the person with active ulcerative colitis, and there is doubt as to whether its occurrence is related to the chronic liver disease associated with ulcerative colitis.

The only physical sign that is occasionally detected is minimal enlargement of the liver. There may be elevated serum transaminase levels.

Pericholangitis

The classical work of Brooke (38) demonstrating portal bacteremia as the cause of pericholangitis remains the best explanation for the genesis of the hepatic inflammation. The characteristic triaditis present in the liver disease of ulcerative colitis has been termed pericholangitis, for in most cases only the portal areas are involved, without the hepatic lobule being affected. A mononuclear infiltrate and enlargement of the portal triad are present initially, without disruption of the limiting plate (Figure 8–2). Later, fibrous deposition occurs, followed by portal-to-portal fibrosis and disruption of the architecture. Cirrhosis follows in some cases.

The clue to the development of pericholangitis is an elevation of the serum alkaline phosphatase. This enzyme becomes markedly elevated, in contrast to almost normal values for transaminases. The elevation in alkaline phosphatase is a direct result of bile duct involvement in the triaditis.

Unless the pericholangitis has progressed to a chronic active hepatitis, to cirrhosis, or to sclerosing cholangitis, there are no symptoms associated with this complication. Mild hepatomegaly can sometimes be detected on physical examination.

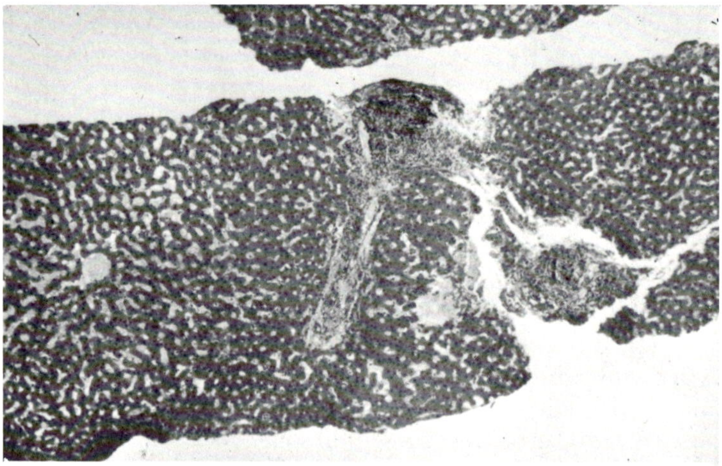

FIGURE 8–2
Liver biopsy specimen showing pericholangitis in a patient with ulcerative colitis. *Above,* low-power photomicrograph. *Below,* high-power view. The inflammatory infiltrate is confined to the portal triad and does not extend into the liver parenchyma (*below, extreme left*).

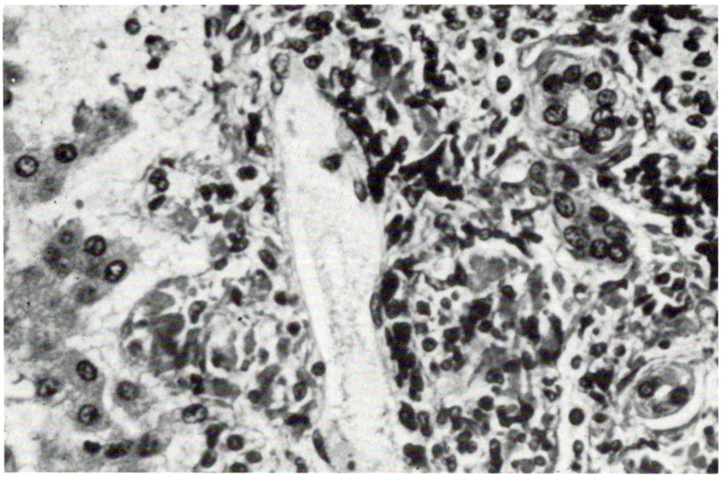

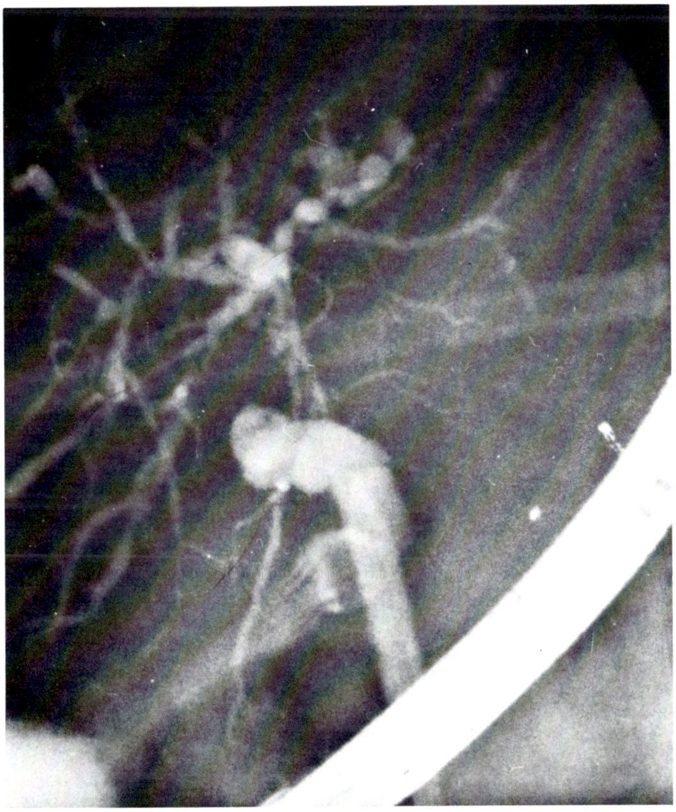

FIGURE 8–3
Endoscopic retrograde cholangiogram demonstrating sclerosing cholangitis in a patient with ulcerative colitis. Note the abnormal beading appearance of the biliary radicles.

Sclerosing Cholangitis

Sclerosing cholangitis is a rare but serious complication of ulcerative colitis. An inflammatory process specifically directed at the bile ducts, especially the larger ducts and in many cases including the extrahepatic ducts, results in their being replaced by fibrous tissue. The ducts become irregularly narrowed, and radiological studies, using endoscopic retrograde cholangiopancreatography (ER CP), show them to have a beaded appearance (Figure 8–3). The process leads to biliary obstruction, to pruritus and jaundice with greatly elevated serum alkaline phosphatase levels, and eventually to cirrhosis. The condition can terminate fatally. A form of surgical bypass is occasionally possible (see Chapter 14).

Chronic Active Hepatitis

Chronic aggressive hepatitis of the nonviral, hepatitis B-negative variety is known to be associated with ulcerative colitis. Either condition can precede the other. In patients with chronic active hepatitis, ulcerative colitis has been known to develop after a number of years. The clinical and pathological picture may have no special features of ulcerative colitis, or there may be an associated pericholangitis. Right upper quadrant abdominal pain is present in the minority of patients; jaundice can occur; other signs, such as splenomegaly, are usually the consequence of a complicating cirrhosis. In most cases, there are no symptoms or physical signs at first, just abnormalities in biochemical liver function tests.

Cirrhosis

If pericholangitis progresses sufficiently, a well-defined cirrhosis occurs, creating a portal cirrhosis similar to primary biliary cirrhosis. Sclerosing cholangitis leads to a similar form of cirrhosis. Chronic active hepatitis also tends to progress to cirrhosis but of a more micronodular type. Unfortunately, the liver disease may be progressive in the face of quiescent ulcerative colitis, so that a cirrhosis may appear without clue or warning.

Postnecrotic cirrhosis secondary to hepatitis B related to blood transfusions also occurs in patients with ulcerative colitis but has a much different appearance. Broad bands of scarring are present in postnecrotic cirrhosis, by comparison with the fine portal cirrhosis of end-stage pericholangitis.

The well-known signs of cirrhosis are intra-abdominal—an enlarged, firm, and often slightly irregular liver, and an enlarged spleen—and extra-abdominal (spider nevi, palmar erythema, etc.).

Bile Duct Carcinoma

Isolated cases of bile duct carcinoma, both intra- and extrahepatic, are being reported with increased frequency in patients with ulcerative colitis. These neoplasms usually arise *de novo;* occasionally there has been preexisting chronic liver disease or pericholangitis. The malignant potential of both the colonic and the bile duct epithelium in ulcerative colitis supports etiological concepts of the hepatobiliary disorders of ulcerative colitis which propose the passage of bacterial products or other antigens in the portal blood from colon to liver.

The majority of patients in whom bile duct carcinoma develops have had total colonic involvement with their colitis. Colectomy does not protect against the development of this malignancy; many cases have been reported to have developed many years after colectomy (39). However, an unanswered question is whether or not colectomy reduces the chances for the development of bile duct carcinoma; there may be a latent period in the genesis of the tumor, and the carcinogenic stimulus may have occurred in earlier years before the colectomy.

Bile duct carcinoma most often presents as an obstructive jaundice. Other symptoms include pain in the right upper quadrant. Irregular enlargement of the liver is a frequent physical sign. However, this tumor is usually unresectable by the time of diagnosis.

Other Hepatobiliary Complications

Secondary amyloidosis and pyogenic liver abscesses have been recorded as hepatic complications of ulcerative colitis. Gallstones appear to be no more frequent among patients with ulcerative colitis than among the general population (unlike the situation in Crohn's disease, in which interruption of the enterohepatic circulation of bile salts by a diseased or resected terminal ileum causes an increased incidence of cholelithiasis); however, gallstones are still probably commoner in patients with ulcerative colitis than are rarities such as sclerosing cholangitis and bile duct carcinoma.

Iatrogenic Liver Disease

Drug-induced liver disease is one of the commonest entities seen by the liver specialist. Patients with ulcerative colitis are liable to be treated with several hepatotoxic drugs, such as chlorpromazine. More specifically, a hepatitis is sometimes seen in patients being treated with azathioprine, which is used in ulcerative colitis. Parenteral hyperalimentation, now being used to treat some cases of refractory ulcerative colitis (see Chapter 13), can be complicated by a fatty liver and elevated serum transaminase levels if too much carbohydrate and insufficient lipid are prescribed.

Diagnosis of the Hepatobiliary Complications

As can be appreciated from the above descriptions, it is difficult to distinguish between the various hepatobiliary complications of ulcerative colitis, and even more difficult to diagnose their presence in the first place. Jaundice, pruritus, and right upper quadrant abdominal pain are the suggestive symptoms. Signs include hepatomegaly and the signs of cirrhosis. Most often, though, there are no symptoms or signs. Patients with ulcerative colitis should have their serum transaminase and alkaline phosphatase levels checked regularly; and if there is any abnormality, or if clinical features suggest hepatobiliary disease even with normal liver function tests, a percutaneous needle liver biopsy should be performed (provided the prothrombin time, the partial thromboplastin time, the bleeding time, and the platelet count are all normal). If the picture is of obstructive jaundice, an important differentiation must be made between sclerosing cholangitis, bile duct carcinoma, and a stone in the common bile duct (and an incidental diagnosis such as carcinoma of the head of the pancreas).

Investigative techniques now available include ultrasonography to detect disorders of the bile ducts (the technique is noninvasive but probably not sufficiently specific to differentiate all the possibilities if the bile ducts are confirmed to be obstructed); skinny-needle percutaneous transhepatic cholangiography (the Chiba technique—in sclerosing cholangitis it may not be possible to enter a bile radicle); and endoscopic retrograde cholangiopancreatography (ERCP), which is probably the most specific for the range of bile duct disorders complicating ulcerative colitis. An exploratory operation may be the only means of making a diagnosis and treating the disorder (see Chapter 14).

When a patient with chronic ulcerative colitis is found to have a disorder of liver function, a liver biopsy may be unnecessary or may be interpreted more accurately if a previous biopsy specimen has been taken and can be compared. The authors suggest that whenever an intra-abdominal operative procedure is performed on a patient with ulcerative colitis, such as a colectomy, the surgeon should perform a wedge liver biopsy for future reference; this is considerably safer than a percutaneous liver biopsy. He should at least report on the macroscopic appearance of the liver surface.

THROMBOEMBOLISM

Deep venous thrombosis and pulmonary embolism may occur in any severe, debilitating disease requiring long periods of bed rest; yet the incidence of phlebitis in ulcerative colitis does appear to be increased beyond that in many other chronic diseases. There may be a hypercoagulable state in ulcerative colitis—increases in the platelet count and the levels of factors V and VIII and fibrinogen have been demonstrated (40). Superficial thrombophlebitis of the leg veins is also seen in patients with ulcerative colitis.

In addition to peripheral venous disorders, thrombosis of cerebral and portal veins has been reported, and also benign intracranial hypertension (which is probably due to cerebral venous obstruction).

Prevention of venous stagnation in patients with ulcerative colitis is important. Patients in bed with active colitis or following surgery should be instructed to perform frequent dorsiflexion of the feet; early ambulation is advisable; and stockings may be needed. These maneuvers are particularly important following total colectomy when the patient has been in a lithotomy position for a long time.

KIDNEY DISORDERS

Despite hypersensitivity reactions in the skin and eyes, these processes do not appear to affect the glomeruli in ulcerative colitis. The only major renal complication of ulcerative colitis is nephrolithiasis, a complication that is probably secondary to disordered physiology in the colon. Acute renal failure has been known to follow a disastrous hemorrhage and is, unfortunately, not an uncommon complication of surgery, particularly a hurried colectomy.

The incidence of kidney stones in patients with ulcerative colitis is roughly twice that in the normal population. Following colectomy and ileostomy, the incidence increases to 20 times normal. The incidence of each of the three major types of urinary tract stone—triple (calcium-magnesium-ammonium) phosphate, calcium oxalate, and uric acid—is greater than normal, but the occurrence of uric acid stones increases more markedly than the other types (41). Oxalate stones, particularly common in Crohn's disease because of a mechanism related to malabsorption of bile salts from the terminal ileum, do not increase in frequency in ulcerative colitis more than the triple phosphate stones.

Although several mechanisms have been proposed for the genesis of kidney stones in ulcerative colitis, the best explanation remains that of straightforward chronic dehydration, especially when the patient has had a colectomy and is left with an ileostomy. There is some evidence that patients with diarrhea from ulcerative colitis become acidotic, as also do patients with an ileostomy (the latter probably more so); this may explain the particular increase in the occurrence of uric acid stones, which are less soluble in acid than in alkali.

Prevention of nephrolithiasis is mainly effected by always ensuring adequate hydration in patients with ulcerative colitis and in patients with an ileostomy. Further aspects of the management of these calculi are discussed in Chapter 14.

ANEMIA

Anemia is very common in patients with ulcerative colitis and can be due to a variety of reversible causes, including hemolysis and deficiencies of iron and folic acid. It is a complication that is most often secondary to disordered colonic pathology (iron deficiency) but may also be part of a systemic disorder (hemolysis) or consequent upon the use of certain drugs (sulfasalazine, azathioprine).

Iron Deficiency

The most common form of anemia in ulcerative colitis is that due to iron loss with inadequate replacement. In addition to the loss of gross blood, the patient continues to lose occult blood for some time after the disease begins to respond to therapy. If iron stores were depleted before the onset of the attack of ulcerative colitis (e.g., following heavy menstruation), then iron deficiency anemia can occur with relatively mild ulcerative colitis. Anorexia or a therapeutic diet forbidding fresh vegetables may have resulted in an inadequate iron intake. The anemia is typically hypochromic and microcytic, but measurement of the serum iron and total iron-binding capacity is essential as the first step in the investigation of any patient with ulcerative colitis and anemia. If iron deficiency is not present, then the more unusual causes of anemia should be sought, such as hemolytic anemia or folic acid deficiency.

Although oral iron replacement is the simplest and best method of therapy, many iron preparations are poorly tolerated by patients with ulcerative colitis, particularly during active phases of the disease. Treatment of the iron deficiency is dealt with in Chapter 13.

Hemolysis

An unusual cause of anemia in ulcerative colitis is an autoimmune hemolytic anemia associated with splenomegaly and a positive Coombs' test (42). The hemolytic anemia is often accompanied by other hypersensitivity phenomena, especially arthritis, and usually responds to corticosteroids.

A more common cause of hemolysis is sulfasalazine therapy. This drug appears to be capable of causing hemolysis due to glucose-6-phosphate deficiency and also (and more commonly) directly and unrelated to any known enzymatic defect within the red cell (43). Hemolysis due to sulfasalazine is so common that it should be suspected in every patient with ulcerative colitis who becomes or remains anemic out of proportion to blood loss and with a normal value for serum iron.

Folic Acid Deficiency

Bland diets sometimes prescribed for or taken voluntarily by patients with ulcerative colitis are somewhat folate-deficient, so that patients who have been on such diets for months without adequate replacement of folic acid may develop a megaloblastic anemia due to folic acid deficiency. Only small amounts of folic acid are required, but several factors can upset this subtle balance, including a demand for more folate by increased erythropoiesis from either recent blood loss or hemolysis. Finally, sulfasalazine has been shown to decrease folic acid absorption from the small intestine (44).

Other Causes of Megaloblastic Anemia

Vitamin B_{12} deficiency is not a feature of ulcerative colitis. The minimal inflammation that can occur in the terminal ileum in "backwash ileitis" is insufficient to interfere significantly with the absorption of vitamin B_{12} in the terminal ileum. If a megaloblastic anemia in ulcerative colitis is found to be due to low serum B_{12} levels or if there is an abnormal Schilling test for B_{12} absorption, the alternative diagnosis of Crohn's disease is a strong possibility. The incidental occurrence of gastric achlorhydria causing vitamin B_{12} malabsorption is quite unusual.

Patients with chronic liver disease associated with ulcerative colitis are liable to develop a macrocytic anemia that is believed to be due to poor folic acid utilization.

Marrow Suppression

The "anemia of chronic disease," due to poor bone marrow activity associated with chronic disease, occurs relatively rarely in ulcerative colitis, usually secondary to malnutrition. Most cases of anemia in patients with ulcerative colitis in whom the red cell indices are normal prove to be due to sulfasalazine-induced hemolysis. Hypoplasia and aplasia of the bone marrow, affecting red cell, white cell, and platelet precursors (though not always each of these equally), are apt to follow the use of azathioprine and, rarely, sulfasalazine. Azathioprine-induced bone marrow suppression is usually reversible; deaths have occurred in patients with ulcerative colitis developing agranulocytosis secondary to sulfasalazine therapy.

OTHER SYSTEMIC COMPLICATIONS

Vasculitis

A systemic vasculitis, with inflammation of the small blood vessels leading to areas of cutaneous necrosis and occasionally pulmonary and renal complications, has been described in association with definite ulcerative colitis (45). In some cases of an apparent association between a systemic vasculitis and ulcerative colitis, it is the vasculitis that is primary and involves the small vessels supplying the colonic mucosa, giving rise to a colitis that is not histologically the condition we call "ulcerative colitis."

Pulmonary Disorders

A few well-documented cases of interstitial pulmonary fibrosis and pulmonary vasculitis have been reported in association with ulcerative colitis (46); and in a recent study a group of patients with ulcerative colitis and Crohn's disease were shown to have poorer pulmonary carbon monoxide transfer than a group of controls (47). Also, sulfasalazine therapy is known to cause a form of pulmonary fibrosis. Patients in whom pericarditis develops in association with ulcerative colitis (see below) often also develop pleural effusions.

Venous thrombosis associated with ulcerative colitis can lead to pulmonary embolism and infarction and to pulmonary hypertension.

There is also a definite increase in the incidence of hay fever and asthma among patients with ulcerative colitis (48).

Cardiac Disorders

The authors and others have reported cases of pericarditis and myocarditis occurring in association with ulcerative colitis; in many but not all instances, these disorders paralleled exacerbations of the colitis, and often occurred concurrently with other extracolonic manifestations of the disease of a "hypersensitivity" type, such as erythema nodosum (49). The authors are currently reviewing the electrocardiograms of their patients with ulcerative colitis and are finding a significant incidence of nonspecific ST and T wave abnormalities, although some of the abnormal findings appear to be due to potassium deficiency.

"Hypersensitivity" myopericarditis must not be confused with right ventricular strain secondary to pulmonary embolization. A lung scan should be performed in any patient with ulcerative colitis who develops an electrocardiographic abnormality.

Thyroid Disorders

There is a definite increased incidence of goiter and thyrotoxicosis in patients with ulcerative colitis, possibly due to the loss of thyroid-bound serum proteins into the feces (50).

Complications Secondary to the Colonic Pathology

Besides blood losses leading to iron deficiency anemia, the inflammation of the colon in ulcerative colitis causes abnormal losses of water, sodium, potassium, and nutrients, especially protein. Dehydration, sodium depletion, and hypokalemia are frequent results, as are malnutrition and growth retardation in children and adolescents (the latter are discussed in Chapter 18). Symptoms related to these secondary systemic effects were described in the last section of Chapter 5. Because ulcerative colitis does not involve the small intestine, hypocalcemia is not a feature, although serum calcium levels may be lowered in parallel with hypoalbuminemia.

III

The Diagnosis

9 DIFFERENTIAL DIAGNOSIS

The diagnosis of ulcerative colitis is suggested by the symptoms described in Chapter 5, by the signs referred to in Chapter 6, and occasionally by symptoms or signs of extracolonic manifestations of the disease as discussed in Chapter 8. The occurrence of one or more of the major symptoms of ulcerative colitis with one of the more common extracolonic symptoms (such as erythema nodosum or ankylosing spondylitis) should point the diagnosis clearly towards ulcerative colitis. The clinical diagnosis is confirmed by means of endoscopy, biopsy, and radiology, as will be described in Chapters 11 and 12. When patients present solely with symptoms of intestinal disease (as do the majority of patients with ulcerative colitis), one can never be sure of the diagnosis, even with the most typical of histories and physical signs. In the investigation of patients complaining of rectal bleeding, diarrhea, abdominal pain, or rectal discomfort, one must be aware not merely of the possibility of ulcerative colitis but also of alternative diagnoses, since such an awareness will ensure the greatest scrutiny of the endoscopic, pathological, and radiological appearances that will come to light as a result of the corresponding investigative procedures.

The diseases that can present similarly to ulcerative colitis fall into two broad groups: those with and those without areas of diffuse inflammation of the colonic mucosa. The former are forms of "colitis" in the true pathological sense of that word. The latter (such as tumors and hemorrhoids) are easier to differentiate from ulcerative colitis, since endoscopy, biopsy, and radiology should always show there to be a normal mucosa except in the region of a local lesion.

DISEASES THAT ARE NOT FORMS OF COLITIS

Diseases that are not forms of colitis are easier to exclude in the differential diagnosis than are the forms of colitis that are not ulcerative colitis (which are the subject of the latter part of this chapter).

Four important conditions, each considerably more common than ulcerative colitis (at least, in the over-40 age group), present with one or more of the same symptoms as ulcerative colitis. These are hemorrhoids, the irritable colon syndrome, diverticular disease, and carcinoma of the colon.

Diverticular Disease and Carcinoma of the Colon

Carcinoma of the colon, quite commonly (always, if untreated), and diverticular disease, rather uncommonly, can be fatal. Both of these conditions can and usually do present with one or more of the four major symptoms of ulcerative colitis: rectal bleeding, diarrhea, abdominal pain, and rectal discomfort. All physicians (and, it is to be hoped, many lay people) know that lives can be saved by the early diagnosis of colonic carcinoma; hence, the investigation of patients suspected of having ulcerative colitis should never be delayed for more than a week or so in case the diagnosis is really carcinoma of the colon.

Both carcinoma of the colon and diverticulosis of the colon are diagnosed by the same means as ulcerative colitis (endoscopy, biopsy, radiology); so there is usually no difficulty in making these diagnoses once those studies have been ordered and carried out competently. Difficulties arise when ulcerative colitis is itself complicated by colonic carcinoma (see Chapter 7). Diverticulosis is uncommonly associated with ulcerative colitis—there seem to be etiological reasons for this, related to the disturbed colonic motor activity in ulcerative colitis. It should be recalled that diverticulosis of the colon is itself so common in the Western world that, if detected on barium X-ray examination, it should not be assumed to be the cause of symptoms of colonic disease unless other diseases have been satisfactorily excluded. Diverticulitis and colonic carcinoma are often accompanied by a mild colitis in an adjacent area (rarely extending more than 3 cm from the local lesion).

Hemorrhoids and the Irritable Colon Syndrome

The symptoms of hemorrhoids are rectal discomfort and rectal bleeding that is bright red and easily confused with the bleeding observed in ulcerative proctitis. Hemorrhoids do not cause diarrhea or abdominal pain. The irritable colon syndrome, on the other hand, causes diarrhea, abdominal pain, or constipation, or any combination of these; but it never causes rectal bleeding. The irritable colon syndrome is totally benign, and hemorrhoids cause only local trouble (except in the rare instance when iron deficiency anemia results from the chronic blood loss). Both conditions can affect young adults, as well as the elderly, and they are both so common that they are often seen simultaneously; possibly the combination of these two disorders occurs more often than ulcerative colitis itself.

Diarrhea

The differential diagnosis of diarrhea includes all the diseases of the small intestine, ranging from the serious, such as celiac sprue, to the common but less serious, such as hypolactasia; postgastrectomy states (for which there should be an adequate history); diseases of the pancreas; hepatobiliary disorders (though these should be apparent on clinical examination and liver function tests); motility disorders of the gastrointestinal tract, such as scleroderma; other gastrointestinal tumors (villous adenoma, carcinoid); hormonal causes, such as thyrotoxicosis; some other diseases (e.g., pneumatosis coli); and drug-induced causes, including digoxin overdosage and laxative abuse. In patients with diarrhea, small bowel disease should always be excluded by performing an upper gastrointestinal and small bowel barium X-ray series, as well as a barium enema X-ray examination. Biochemical and hematological parameters such as hypocalcemia, hypocholestrolemia, and vitamin B_{12} deficiency may point to small intestinal disease.

Hypolactasia

The most common diarrheal "illness" in the world, statistically, is primary intestinal lactase deficiency, if such a prevalent condition can be called an illness. Actually, in terms of the world population, the ability to digest lactose, although normal in European man, is the abnormal condition. It is a condition of significance only in societies (like the Western) in which people over the age of 2 years consume cow's milk and dairy products. Since lactose intolerance is so common, it frequently coexists with ulcerative colitis, producing a confusing picture. Patients with hypolactasia do have more severe attacks of ulcerative colitis (23). Lactose intolerance should not be confused with true milk allergy, which is mainly a condition of young children.

The simplest way to diagnose lactose intolerance is to perform a lactose tolerance test. Alternatively, if the patient gives a clear history of milk intolerance, a therapeutic trial of a lactose-free diet should be introduced for several weeks. If the diarrhea does not improve appreciably, milk should be cautiously reintroduced to see if diarrhea, gas pains, or urgency worsen. Since milk is an excellent source of protein, calcium, and fat, this useful nutritional product should not be needlessly restricted and a lactose challenge should always be performed after several weeks of apparent improvement on a lactose-free diet if a lactose tolerance test was not done initially.

Rectal Bleeding

The differential diagnosis of rectal bleeding (in the noncolitis group of disorders) includes benign colonic polyps; angiodysplastic lesions in the colonic mucosa (most commonly on the right side of the colon, and often found in elderly patients suffering from heart disease); and hematological disorders, including leukemic and lymphomatous involvement of the rectum, coagulopathies, and overdosage with anticoagulant drugs. The coagulopathies are diagnosed by appropriate hematological investigations, whereas the other diseases listed here as causing rectal bleeding are diagnosed mainly by endoscopy (colonoscopy more often than sigmoidoscopy).

Abdominal Pain

Abdominal pain can be caused by any of the conditions mentioned above which can give rise to diarrhea. Other conditions that give rise to abdominal pain which enter into the differential diagnosis of ulcerative colitis include acute appendicitis; the various causes of intestinal obstruction; gallbladder disease; renal and ureteric pain from calculi or from pyelonephritis; and gynecological disorders such as salpingitis. In the investigation of abdominal pain, the patient's history and the findings of the physical examination are extremely important, but to exclude diagnoses of these conditions, it is usually necessary to request a cholecystogram and an intravenous pyelogram and to perform a gynecological examination.

FORMS OF COLITIS OTHER THAN ULCERATIVE COLITIS

Diseases (other than ulcerative colitis) that can give rise to mucosal inflammation in the colon are included under this heading. In some of them (e.g., Crohn's disease), the inflammation can, in fact, be confined to the small intestine; but in these instances the symptoms of rectal bleeding, diarrhea, and abdominal pain can still occur. There are some clinical features that help to identify diseases in this group; but a firm diagnosis is made by means of sigmoidoscopy or colonoscopy, often together with biopsy, to confirm the differentiation from ulcerative colitis, and by means of barium enema X-ray examination. A barium meal and small bowel follow-through X-ray series is important in identifying Crohn's disease involving the small intestine.

The forms of colitis other than ulcerative colitis divide themselves into those that are acute diseases and those that are chronic diseases. When a patient presents acutely in a first attack of ulcerative colitis, both the acute and chronic forms of colitis enter into the differential diagnosis, whereas when a patient gives a history suggestive of chronic ulcerative colitis, the differential diagnosis does not include the forms of colitis that are always acute (except in the situation where there is a sudden worsening of symptoms compatible with a new acute disease following on a more chronic and unrelated condition, such as hemorrhoidal bleeding).

The pathological features of these other forms of colitis were described in Chapter 4. Their endoscopic and radiological features will be alluded to in Chapters 11 and 12, respectively. In the remainder of this chapter, some clinical points that suggest an alternative form of colitis to ulcerative colitis will be mentioned.

Acute Forms of Colitis

Acute Infections

Of the various bacterial and viral acute infections that cause gastroenteritis and colitis, the common forms that last one to three days are now believed to be caused by viruses (rotaviruses) and by toxigenic strains of *Escherichia coli.* These cause diarrhea, occasionally accompanied by rectal bleeding.

Usually more severe and lasting as long as one to two weeks is *Shigella* dysentery. Since this condition generally does cause rectal bleeding, it is more likely to be confused with an acute first attack of ulcerative colitis than infections with rotaviruses or *E. coli.* In fact, the sigmoidoscopic and biopsy features of shigellosis may be indistinguishable from those of ulcerative colitis, and the diagnosis relies on stool culture, which should be performed on every new case of suspected ulcerative colitis, particularly when the patient has a history of travel in a hot country.

Salmonella infections include gastroenteritis and paratyphoid, which cause an acute diarrheal illness often with colonic involvement, and typhoid fever, which is more a debilitating febrile illness in which bloody diarrhea only comes on in the second week of the disease.

Protozoal forms of gastrointestinal infection (such as amebiasis and giardiasis) can become chronic and are therefore considered in the differential diagnosis of chronic colitis (below).

Yersinia enterocolitica causes an acute bacterial infection that principally affects the terminal ileum and closely resembles an acute attack of Crohn's disease. It can also cause inflammation of the colon, appreciated as a colitis on sigmoidoscopy or colonoscopy, frequently with aphthoid ulcers. Even when there is a colitis, radiology shows the main lesion to be a terminal ileitis. Rectal biopsy specimens show features overlapping those both of ulcerative colitis and of Crohn's disease. A peripheral polyarthritis can complicate the picture, and this can be especially suggestive of inflammatory bowel disease. The clinical course lasts one to four weeks. Specific diagnosis is by culture of the stool; it is helpful to determine *Y. enterocolitica* serum antibody titers (51).

Membranous Colitis

Membranous (or pseudomembranous) colitis nowadays generally occurs following the use of broad-spectrum antibiotics, particularly lincomycin and clindamycin. A few cases are due to staphylococcal overgrowth following suppression of other components of the bowel flora by the antibiotic, but the cause of most cases is unknown; a viral etiology has been suggested. The condition can also be seen without previous antibiotic administration, following severe hypoxia or hypotension. Hence, it is a complication of abdominal and thoracic surgical procedures. Membranous colitis follows an acute course lasting up to a few weeks, but it is not a recurrent condition. Otherwise its clinical presentation may be identical to that of ulcerative colitis, although profuse mucus diarrhea is a frequent feature.

Vascular Causes of Colitis

Ischemic colitis and other types of mesenteric vascular disease can mimic ulcerative colitis. Like membranous colitis (which etiologically may also be a form of vascular insufficiency), these conditions last a few days to a few weeks but are rarely recurrent. They mostly give rise to gastrointestinal bleeding out of proportion to any diarrhea they may cause. Ischemic colitis itself is most common in elderly persons; it generally causes a segmental form of colitis—most often at the splenic flexure where the supplies of the superior and inferior mesenteric arteries abut on each other with poor collaterals; it is fairly acute, and may heal with the formation of a colonic stricture. Cases of segmental colitis are seen in young persons, often affecting the right side of the colon, and most commonly in women taking the contraceptive pill.

Mesenteric embolism with intestinal infarction is a catastrophic condition, with hemorrhage, diarrhea, abdominal pain, and shock, which must be distinguished from fulminant ulcerative colitis. Physical examination may reveal a source for an embolus (e.g., mitral stenosis), or the patient may have a history of ischemic cardiovascular disease; and a plain abdominal X-ray film may show a paralytic ileus or air in the submucosa of the intestine (a form of pneumatosis intestinalis). Mesenteric vein thrombosis can produce a similar picture. Chronic mesenteric arterial insufficiency is more likely to cause severe recurrent abdominal pain.

Chronic Forms of Colitis

Protozoal Infections

Amebiasis is one of the hardest conditions to differentiate from ulcerative colitis. On clinical grounds it may be impossible, although knowledge that the patient has traveled in a tropical country may be helpful to the physician. The symptoms are really no different from those of ulcerative colitis. The diagnosis is made by microscopic examination of a *fresh* stool (best obtained at sigmoidoscopy) and by observation of certain sigmoidoscopic features (Chapter 11) and by biopsy.

Rarer protozoal infections that can involve the colon are the infection caused by *Balantidium coli,* which is clinically similar to amebiasis though it more often affects the right side of the colon, and schistosomiasis, which most often affects the rectum and distal colon.

Giardia lamblia causes a protozoal infection of the gastrointestinal tract that is generally subacute or chronic. It produces diarrhea, and it involves the small intestine rather than the large intestine, causing malabsorption. There is no significant colonic inflammation. The infection does not cause rectal bleeding, but anemia may result from the malabsorptive state. Knowledge that the patient has traveled in certain known endemic areas (the most well-known currently being Leningrad) helps in pointing to the diagnosis. The diagnosis is made by microscopic examination of the stool or of a duodenal aspirate.

Viral, Bacterial, and Fungal Infections

Other infections in which the colon may be affected include lymphogranuloma venereum, which nearly always is accompanied by other clinical evidence of perineal infection with the *Bedsonia* virus; gonorrhea, which causes a gonococcal proctitis most commonly seen in male homosexuals and is diagnosed by rectal cultures, as well as by the usual urethral and cervical cultures; tuberculosis, which can affect the rectum, causing chronic fissured ulcers similar to those in Crohn's disease; and the fungal diseases histoplasmosis and candidiasis, seen particularly in patients receiving immunosuppressant or antitumor drugs.

Radiation Colitis

Radiation colitis and enteritis can be confused with ulcerative colitis. A good clue is the patient's history of having received therapeutic irradiation, most commonly for uterine or cervical carcinoma. Radiation enteritis affects the small intestine, causing malabsorption, diarrhea, and fairly typical changes that can be seen on a small bowel X-ray series. Radiation proctitis more often mimics ulcerative colitis; occasionally an acute proctitis occurs in the weeks following the radiotherapy, but usually it arises a few years later. The patient complains of rectal bleeding, sometimes accompanied by diarrhea. The bleeding may be scanty and is often accompanied by mucus; at times the bleeding is very heavy. Characteristically, the bleeding is intermittent, with months without symptoms, and then a torrential bleed occurs. The sigmoidoscopic features resemble some of those in ulcerative colitis (for instance, the granularity); however, a rectal biopsy (see Chapter 4) confirms a suspicion of radiation proctitis.

Solitary Rectal Ulcer Syndrome

The solitary rectal ulcer syndrome (52) is a condition that causes rectal bleeding, mucus discharge, and rectal discomfort. It is mainly a disease of women in their 20s. Its features can be identified sigmoidoscopically as a solitary granular ulcerated area in the rectum, and the pathology can be confirmed with a biopsy (see Chapter 4). This syndrome is a chronic indolent condition. Because it is relatively rare and occurs in the same age group as does ulcerative colitis, many patients with this condition are told they have ulcerative colitis, which is incorrect. It never progresses beyond the rectum; it usually improves as the patient gets older; and surgery should almost never be required.

Behçet's Disease

Behçet's disease can ulcerate the anus and rectum, as well as the mouth and the genital mucosa. The syndrome also includes uveitis and arthritis and frequently thrombophlebitis, which can cause confusion with the extracolonic manifestations of ulcerative colitis. The inflammation of the rectum tends to be more patchy and indurated and the ulcers deeper than in ulcerative colitis.

Crohn's Disease

The etiological, epidemiological, pathological, clinical, endoscopic, and radiological features of Crohn's disease are very close to those of ulcerative colitis, as discussed in Chapters 2, 3, 4, 8, 11, and 12, and many aspects of treatment are similar. Ulcerative colitis and Crohn's disease are often referred to together as *inflammatory bowel disease.* Clinical differentiation of the two conditions is important because Crohn's disease is apt to involve the small intestine (and also the duodenum, the stomach, and the mouth). This means that a total colectomy operation is not necessarily curative for Crohn's disease of the colon, as it would be for ulcerative colitis. There are other differences; for instance, the much lower incidence of carcinoma of the colon in Crohn's disease. Hence, the gastroenterologist has a duty to decide whether a patient with inflammatory bowel disease has ulcerative colitis or Crohn's disease, and this requires an open mind at all times and constant reevaluation. There are a few cases that seem to be truly on the border line, showing features of both conditions. Nevertheless, this said, the diagnosis of inflammatory bowel disease can be a sufficient working diagnosis in an acute phase, since the therapy for an acute attack of both diseases is more or less the same, especially when the Crohn's disease involves considerable segments of the large intestine.

Pathological differences between ulcerative colitis and Crohn's disease were discussed in Chapter 4, and the endoscopic and radiological differences will be described in Chapters 11 and 12. A patient with any of the clinical presentations of ulcerative colitis, including any of the systemic complications of ulcerative colitis, might be suffering from Crohn's disease. There are, on the other hand, a number of clinical features that are specific for Crohn's disease rather than ulcerative colitis. These are as follows: an inflammatory mass in the abdomen, usually in the right lower quadrant; malabsorption, particularly of calcium and vitamin B_{12}; intestinal obstruction, either acute or intermittent; involvement of the duodenum, the stomach, or the mouth with inflammatory bowel disease; fistulas from the bowel into other parts of the bowel, into the bladder or the vagina, or through the skin; and severe perianal disease with fissures, fistulas, and abscesses. The reader is referred to the companion book in this series, *Crohn's Disease* by Drs. Schachter and Kirsner (53).

Factitious Proctitis

Finally, it should not be forgotten that there are persons who, as a result of psychiatric peculiarities, insert instruments or unusual fluids into the rectum, sometimes as part of deviant sexual practices, sometimes to initiate medical investigations (corresponding to the Munchausen syndrome). Traumatic rectal ulcers result, with the remainder of the mucosa being entirely normal. Such patients require skillful handling by the physician and a psychiatrist.

10

EVALUATION OF THE PATIENT

The evaluation of the patient known or suspected to have ulcerative colitis consists of confirming the diagnosis and then assessing the severity of the disease and noting the presence of any local or systemic complications. Once the patient's history has been taken and the physical examination performed, the initial investigation should always include the following: a complete blood count (for hemoglobin, hematocrit, red cell indexes, white cell count and differential counts) and an examination of the red cell morphology and measurement of the sedimentation rate; a multiple channel biochemical screen, including tests for blood urea and electrolytes, creatinine, bilirubin, transaminases, alkaline phosphatase, calcium, albumin, total protein, cholesterol, and uric acid; stool cultures for *Shigella* and *Salmonella* organisms and microscopy of the fresh stool for the causative organisms of amebiasis and giardiasis; urine analysis; a rectal examination; a vaginal examination; sigmoidoscopy; and either a barium enema X-ray examination (or a firsthand review of a very recent and completely performed barium enema study) or, when the disease is moderately or severely active, a plain abdominal X-ray, with the barium enema X-ray examination postponed for a few weeks until the patient's condition is quiescent.

The presence of leukocytes in the stool is a feature of active ulcerative colitis but is also common in many other forms of colonic inflammation and is therefore not specific; detection of such leukocytes may be a useful screening test for colonic disease for the general practitioner, but the authors have not found it helpful in gastroenterological practice.

A *Salmonella* serum agglutination test should be sought if infection with this species is a possibility, especially if the patient has recently traveled in hot and unhygienic areas.

An electrocardiogram and a chest X-ray film should be ordered (or recent studies should be available) for patients with more than a mild distal colitis in case an urgent decision for surgery has to be made.

If there is the slightest doubt about the diagnosis, the sigmoidoscopy should be accompanied by a rectal biopsy; see Chapter 11 for a discussion of the indications for rectal biopsy and also for the place of colonoscopy.

It is a good idea for the patient to have an upper gastrointestinal barium X-ray series together with a small bowel follow-through X-ray series at some stage; this helps to exclude Crohn's disease and other small intestinal disorders, and it also allows the detection of other esophageal, gastric, and small bowel diseases that might otherwise be overlooked and that might confuse the clinical picture. For example, in evaluating abdominal pain or a particularly heavy gastrointestinal hemorrhage, it is important to know about the presence of a gastric or duodenal ulcer. The upper gastrointestinal barium X-ray series is conveniently combined with a gallbladder X-ray study. When the urinalysis is abnormal or if the blood urea or creatinine is elevated, or if there is anything in the history or in the plain abdominal X-ray film to suggest urinary tract disease, an intravenous pyelogram should be performed.

Systemic complications (such as those of the joints, the liver, or the eyes) may require further evaluation, as described in Chapter 8.

MILD, MODERATE, AND SEVERE ULCERATIVE COLITIS

Besides making a firm diagnosis of ulcerative colitis, the physician must assess the severity of activity of the disease and the extent of the involvement of the colon. The extent of the colitis is most conveniently assessed by barium enema X-ray examination; colonoscopy will also show the extent and tends to reveal more widespread disease than is apparent on barium enema X-ray examination. It is also important to ascertain the year in which the colitis probably began, taking this as when the patient first had suggestive symptoms.

In the discussion in Chapter 13 on the medical treatment of ulcerative colitis, the terms *mild, moderate,* and *severe* will be used to designate grades of severity. It is also acceptable to use intermediate grades—very mild, mild-to-moderate, moderate-to-severe—and the most severe forms of the disease can be considered *fulminant.* These grades of severity can be assigned on the basis of sigmoidoscopic appearances, radiological appearances, and the clinical picture of the patient, and also by studying the rectal biopsy specimen (the latter is useful for blind assessment of activity in drug trials). In practice, the authors grade patients according to the clinical picture and the sigmoidoscopic features, but the barium enema X-ray study does help. The sigmoidoscopic classification is described in Chapter 11.

The presence of fever, weight loss, hemorrhage lowering the hematocrit to below 30%, a low plasma albumin level, diarrhea more than five or six times daily, or troublesome extracolonic manifestations is an indication that the disease is in at least the moderate category. When these features are marked (e.g., a temperature of 39°C, or more than 12 stools in twenty-four hours), or when more than two or three of them are present at once, one can say there is severe disease. With none of these features, the clinical picture is that of mild disease. Because ulcerative colitis is not considered to remit completely from a biological point of view, the term *quiescent* colitis can be applied to patients who, having suffered an attack of the disease, no longer have any symptoms.

In the next two chapters, the endoscopic and radiological features of ulcerative colitis will be described. When performing endoscopic and radiological studies, it should be borne in mind that their role is to evaluate the severity of the disease, as well as to make or confirm the diagnosis.

11

ENDOSCOPY AND BIOPSY

SIGMOIDOSCOPY

Sigmoidoscopy is the single most valuable diagnostic study in ulcerative colitis because it permits direct visualization of the mucosa of the rectum and the sigmoid colon. In early or mild ulcerative colitis, the results of the barium enema X-ray examination are frequently normal, so that the proctosigmoidoscopic examination is the only objective means of diagnosis. Sigmoidoscopy should be part of the routine physical examination in every patient with rectal bleeding. It is the fastest and surest way to diagnose (or to exclude) ulcerative colitis; and other important causes of rectal bleeding (such as carcinoma or Crohn's disease in the rectosigmoid) can be diagnosed in this way. The procedure also affords the possibility of taking a biopsy of the rectal mucosa (see below).

Depth of Examination

"Sigmoidoscopy" is the examination of the rectum and the sigmoid colon using a rigid tubular instrument (metal or plastic). The conventional sigmoidoscope is 30 cm in length, and the examination of the rectosigmoid is normally performed to the length of the instrument, if this is possible without damaging the mucosa or causing undue pain. However, in patients with ulcerative colitis an examination of such depth is often unnecessary and may be actually unwise. In active colitis the examination may be very painful, and if the rectum is seen to be inflamed, there is no need to proceed beyond a depth of 10 to 15 cm to make the diagnosis. In fact, in a patient with ulcerative colitis the examination should only be attempted beyond 10 to 15 cm in the following situations:

1. To determine the upper limit of involvement with colitis when the rectum is seen to be involved but when there is a possibility that the disease is limited to the rectosigmoid. Previous X-ray evidence of more extensive disease (seen by barium enema X-ray examination or in plain abdominal film X-ray by loss of colonic haustrations) or previous sigmoidoscopic or colonoscopic evidence of disease beyond a depth of 30 cm excludes the possibility of limited disease, as does a fulminating clinical course, in which a deep sigmoidoscopic examination is unwarranted.

2. To diagnose the severity of ulcerative colitis when there is rectal sparing or when it is suspected that there is more severe involvement of the sigmoid than of the rectum.

3. To exclude carcinoma in the rectosigmoid. A sigmoidoscopic examination to a depth of 30 cm should be attempted by the physician *a*) when the first attack he has observed has become quiescent; *b*) when a patient who has had ulcerative colitis for more than five years suffers a relapse of symptoms; and *c*) at least once every six months in a patient who has had ulcerative colitis for more than seven years (see Chapter 15).

Patients in whom the sigmoidoscopy reveals a severely inflamed rectum should not be examined beyond a depth of 10 to 12 cm until there are clinical signs of a response to treatment of the acute attack.

"Proctoscopy"

The term "proctoscopy" is confusing. In Britain it is actually used for the examination which in the United States is called "anoscopy." In America it is used by some physicians alternatively for sigmoidoscopy and by others to refer to a limited sigmoidoscopic examination. In view of this ambiguity, the authors have chosen not to use the term "proctoscopy" in this book. A "sigmoidoscopy" need not be to the full length of the instrument. When it is certain in advance that a sigmoidoscopic examination is to be limited, a short sigmoidoscope of 20 cm or 15 cm in length may be used, although a 30-cm instrument should always be available.

Preparation

In ulcerative colitis of any degree of activity, preparation for sigmoidoscopic examination should be avoided. Many physicians request that the patient have an enema prior to sigmoidoscopy. This is correct in patients without colitis in whom a tumor is being sought, but in patients suspected of having ulcerative colitis an unprepared examination is better, since it allows observation of the natural state of the rectal mucosa unaltered by enemas.

Mild edema and erythema often develop in a normal mucosa after one or two enemas, particularly of the small-volume disposable type; and when more vigorous preparation is used, mild friability may even appear. These changes can also be seen histologically. Phosphate enemas (such as Fleet's) and Dulcolax suppositories and also Dulcolax tablets have been shown to induce such changes. However, physiologically "normal" saline (0.9%) rarely causes these changes and is the preparation of choice if an enema is required in patients with known or suspected ulcerative colitis (54). Since friability of the mucosa seems to be the single best objective sign of ulcerative colitis, the advantages of an unprepared examination can be appreciated. Furthermore, preparatory enemas may make a mild ulcerative colitis appear to be more severe, alarming both the patient and the physician.

Sigmoidoscopy after an enema is often traumatic to the patient with ulcerative colitis since irritability and spasm of the bowel may be present. Many patients with ulcerative colitis have experiences of unpleasant sigmoidoscopic examinations, perhaps by a well-meaning but inexperienced physician; so a simple, unprepared examination comes as a pleasant surprise to the patient, often helping him to establish a positive rapport with the new physician. Finally, since the patient may need to be examined repeatedly, it is much easier and more acceptable to the patient to know that an enema will not be required prior to the examination.

The presence of stool is usually not a problem; for the patient with severe diarrhea generally has a clean rectum, or the mucosa can easily be observed if the soft fecal material is wiped away. In milder disease, the stool is formed and can be bypassed by the sigmoidoscope. The patient with a rectum full of pasty soft stool presents a problem, but the physician can elect to discontinue the examination, to ask the patient to go and try once again to empty his bowel, and then to resume the examination.

Technique

The technique of sigmoidoscopy can only be learned firsthand from an experienced gastroenterologist. General anesthesia should never be required in an adult now that flexible colonoscopy is available for those situations in which, formerly, anesthesia may have been used (in patients with ulcerative colitis, this would only have been to investigate a suspicious tumor at a depth of 15 to 30 cm). Sedation for sigmoidoscopy with 5 to 8 mg of diazepam is acceptable and is sometimes necessary in nervous patients, but in skilled hands the examination should not be too uncomfortable or too prolonged for the majority of patients to forego premedication.

For the examiner, the only points to be emphasized regarding the procedure itself are: 1) Always see the lumen before advancing the instrument, and 2) do not inflict undue pain, and regard the complaint of severe pain by the patient as a sign that there is some reason for obstruction to the passage of the instrument, in which case the examination should be halted. If these two rules are observed, there should be no occurrence of perforation of the bowel by the sigmoidoscope, as does sometimes occur.

Repeated Examinations

Serial examinations serve a useful purpose in allowing assessments of therapy. Such examinations can nearly always be limited to a depth of 10 to 12 cm. An exception to this is the patient treated with local rectal corticosteroids who shows improvement in the rectum yet in whom clinical evidence suggests significant disease more proximally.

SIGMOIDOSCOPIC APPEARANCES

The sigmoidoscopic appearances in ulcerative colitis include acute and chronic abnormalities. The normal rectal mucosa is thin, smooth, pale, and dry, with moderately large blood vessels easily seen through the mucosa. Minimal amounts of mucus may be present. There is no other exudate.

Acute Changes

The earliest abnormalities of ulcerative colitis are edema and erythema, producing a reddened, swollen, and boggy mucosa, often with increased amounts of mucus, so that the vascular pattern can no longer be appreciated. These changes can be seen in any patient with diarrhea and have been called the "diarrhea effect." As the disease becomes more severe, the first distinctive abnormality of friability appears. Friability is defined as contact bleeding, either when the distal edge of the sigmoidoscope abrades the mucosa or when the mucosa is wiped with cotton. This latter maneuver should be done in every patient suspected of having ulcerative colitis. Friability is the sigmoidoscopic hallmark of ulcerative colitis; for even in the most severe cases of noninflammatory diarrhea there should not be contact bleeding.

As the disease becomes acute, spontaneous bleeding and a purulent exudate are seen, so that a sanguinomucopurulent exudate is encountered in the lumen upon inserting the sigmoidoscope. There may be so much of this exudate as to preclude an adequate examination of the rectal wall, but every effort should be made to see the mucosa, such as by wiping or by washing away the exudate with saline. In these instances, the correct impression of severe, active ulcerative colitis is obtained. The most severe changes include frank ulcerations that bleed and exude pus. In a severe initial attack of ulcerative colitis, the mucosa may be diffusely edematous, exuding pus, with diffuse petechial bleeding points.

Chronic Changes

As the acute lesion resolves under therapy, the rectum often returns to normal. If a sufficient amount of mucosal damage has been sustained, often by recurrent acute episodes, then chronic changes appear. These abnormalities include loss of the normal vascular pattern, fine or coarse granularity of the mucosa, hyperplastic polyps (occasionally with mucosal bridging), and some degree of narrowing of the rectal lumen.

Granularity gives the mucosa the appearance of fine or coarse sandpaper, in contrast to the normal smooth glistening surface.

Hyperplastic polyps are created by mucosal inflammation and show large numbers of polymorphonuclear leukocytes histologically. These inflammatory polyps are seen in moderate or severe ulcerative colitis and are also known as pseudopolyps. They represent areas of regenerating mucosa remaining after much of the mucosa has been denuded by an attack of ulcerative colitis. These pseudopolyps persist following resolution of the attack. Mucosal bridging is uncommon and represents two pseudopolyps that have come together to form a bridge. Neither of these polypoid lesions is associated with any premalignant potential.

Rectal luminal stenosis may occur with long-standing disease, even when the disease is localized to the rectum. An associated radiological change as a consequence of luminal narrowing is an increase in the retrorectal or presacral space between the posterior wall of the rectum and the anterior surface of the sacrum.

Detection of Complications

Sigmoidoscopy is important in the detection of carcinoma in patients with long-standing ulcerative colitis; for as many as 40% of such tumors are within reach of the 30-cm sigmoidoscope. Strictures may be within the reach of the sigmoidoscope and may be benign or malignant. Benign strictures are smoother, but all strictures should be subjected to multiple biopsies and cytology.

Ulcerative Proctitis

Ulcerative proctitis is diagnosed only by sigmoidoscopy and represents ulcerative colitis limited to the rectum, with normal mucosa seen above the diseased area. The barium enema X-ray findings are nearly always normal in ulcerative proctitis. Usually the mucosa appears mildly granular and friable, with a moderate amount of mucous exudate and occasionally a little fresh blood.

The important diagnostic feature is the line delineating diseased from normal mucosa; therefore, during the initial sigmoidoscopy, efforts should be made to see an upper border of inflammation, unless the examination becomes too uncomfortable for the patient. In a patient whose symptoms are not compatible with ulcerative proctitis, such as severe bloody diarrhea, there is no need to seek an upper border to the inflammation.

Mild, Moderate, and Severe Ulcerative Colitis

The classification of Truelove (55) is best followed in grading the severity of ulcerative colitis. Mild colitis implies hyperemia, petechiae, and fragility. In moderate colitis these changes are more severe, and there may also be purulent exudates and discrete small ulcers. In severe colitis there is gross pus, spontaneous diffuse bleeding, and a boggy, deep-red mucosa; or there are large areas of ulceration.

In quiescent colitis the only changes that are compatible with the presumed absence of activity are loss of the vascular pattern, minimal hyperemia, or the appearance of the chronic changes described above (narrowing, pseudopolyps).

DIFFERENTIAL DIAGNOSIS (see also Chapter 9)

Noncolitic Disorders

The differentiation of colitis from noncolitic disorders should be easily made on sigmoidoscopy.

Colorectal carcinomas should be apparent as nodules or strictures; they are missed only as a result of an insufficiently deep sigmoidoscopic examination—this, unfortunately, is not an uncommon occurrence.

Endometriosis occasionally resembles a nodular tumor: a biopsy makes the distinction.

Polyps are not overlooked if the sigmoidoscope is withdrawn carefully, complete 360° sweeps being made with the instrument at every level.

Diverticulitis of the sigmoid colon may be appreciated by seeing an area of mild inflammation in relation to a stricture or to the visible opening of a diverticulum.

Perianal lesions (hemorrhoids, fissures, and fistulas) are seen by slowly withdrawing the sigmoidoscope through the anal canal; a supplementary anoscopic examination may be needed.

Diffuse noncolitic lesions include the features of rectal prolapse—an erythematous mucosa that may ulcerate in one or two places and bleed—and laxative abuse, which may cause loss of the vascular pattern, a mild erythema, and sometimes the patchy brown or black crazy-paving effect of melanosis coli.

In the irritable colon syndrome the sigmoidoscopic appearances should be entirely normal; misdiagnosis may be made if a compulsive patient has excessively purged himself with enemas prior to the examination.

Forms of Colitis Other Than Ulcerative Colitis

The differential diagnosis of the group of diseases that are forms of colitis, but not ulcerative colitis, requires careful attention to sigmoidoscopic detail; and often a biopsy is necessary for proof of the diagnosis (see Chapter 4 for the pathological features).

Shigella dysentery may give rise to appearances identical to those of ulcerative colitis, though the hyperemia tends to be more intense and ulceration tends to be more purulent than in ulcerative colitis.

In the common forms of viral and bacterial diarrhea (e.g., in toxigenic *Escherichia coli* infection and paratyphoid), the rectal mucosa may show a mild diffuse colitis, with hyperemia, friability, or granularity; but the infection may be primarily small intestinal, leaving a normal rectal mucosa or one that shows the mild edema and hyperemia of the "diarrhea effect." In *Salmonella typhi* infection there may be lymphoid hyperplasia visible in the rectal mucosa. *Giardia lamblia* infection causes no colitis, only a diarrhea effect.

Amebiasis generally causes discrete ulcerations that are classically flask-shaped, with the neck of the flask towards the lumen. Large ulcers with overhanging edges may be seen; the smaller forms of these ulcers appear as pinpoint ulcerations exuding pus. There may also be a mild diffuse hyperemia. *Balantidium coli* infections may resemble those of amebiasis.

Gonococcal proctitis causes a diffuse or patchy mild inflammation of the rectum that may be indistinguishable from ulcerative proctitis.

The following less common conditions can give rise to limited areas of edematous and indurated rectal inflammation: tuberculosis, lymphogranuloma venereum, histoplasmosis, candidiasis, and leukemic and lymphomatous infiltrations.

Membranous colitis is typified by plaques of adherent white membrane on an intensely red and inflamed and ulcerated colonic mucosa. The surface of the mucosa bleeds when the membrane is pulled off. The membrane may not be seen at all, there simply being a moderate or severe colitis, with much pus and mucus. In milder forms of membranous colitis, the mucosa is just very red, with less friability than in ulcerative colitis.

Ischemic colitis uncommonly involves the rectosigmoid. In the absence of such involvement, the rectal mucosa appears normal. In rare elderly patients and in some younger patients, a diffuse granularity of the mucosa with ulceration may appear; pus is generally not seen.

In acute radiation proctitis there is hyperemic inflammation. In chronic radiation proctitis there is granularity of the mucosa with relatively little hyperemia, and telangiectases may be seen; the mucosa is somewhat atrophic (appreciated better histologically).

The solitary rectal ulcer syndrome describes the appearance of a linear ulcer on the anterior rectal wall, extending from about 5 to 10 cm of sigmoidoscopic depth. The ulcer is surrounded by about one centimeter of erythema and induration, but the remainder of the mucosa usually appears normal.

Features suggesting Crohn's disease rather than ulcerative colitis are the following: a patchy inflammation or rectal sparing; isolated aphthous ulcers; an irregularly edematous mucosa; deep linear ulcers that may become fissured (these latter two features give rise to the typical "cobblestone" appearance); and less friability and granularity of the mucosa than in ulcerative colitis. The presence of pseudopolyps is more typical of ulcerative colitis, but these are not unknown in Crohn's disease. In ulcerative colitis, the inflammation is more evenly diffuse than in Crohn's disease. Perianal fissuring, even with a normal-appearing rectal mucosa, suggests a diagnosis of Crohn's disease rather than ulcerative colitis.

COLONOSCOPY

The fiberoptic colonoscope allows an endoscopic examination of the colon beyond the limits of the rigid sigmoidoscope—as far as the ileocecal valve in many cases. The absolute limit of sigmoidoscopy is the length of the instrument (30 cm) but may be less than this because of difficulties in straightening the rectosigmoid with the rigid instrument. The fiberoptic colonoscope is not needed routinely in ulcerative colitis, but there are particular circumstances in which it can or should be used, particularly in the search for neoplasia.

The preparation for colonoscopy and the examination itself have their risks when performed in active ulcerative colitis. The risks are those of perforation of the acutely inflamed colon and exacerbation of the colitis by the preparative procedures. When the disease is completely inactive, the normal preparation of a few days on a liquid diet followed by aperients and enemas can be undertaken without danger. If mild activity is suspected and the examination is thought to be necessary, then it is generally sufficient to prepare the patient with a liquid diet and physiological saline enemas. In patients with chronic inactive or minimally active ulcerative colitis, the colonoscopic examination is actually safer and easier than in a normal person because of the shortening of the colon and the disappearance of the haustral folds that are characteristic changes in the chronic disease.

The main use of colonoscopy in ulcerative colitis is in the patient with long-standing disease involving most or all of the colon who is a candidate for the development of a carcinoma. By means of colonoscopy, suspicious lesions, previously seen on barium enema X-ray film, such as strictures, areas of irregular mucosa, and isolated or atypical polyps, can be visualized endoscopically; also, and more important, multiple biopsy specimens can be taken from the specific sites of abnormality under direct vision, and the sites can be brushed to collect cells for cytological examination. These procedures can, of course, be done through the rigid sigmoidoscope if the abnormalities are within reach of that instrument, but often they are not.

Whether or not colonoscopy should be performed routinely every 6 or 12 months in patients who have had ulcerative colitis more than seven years is a debatable point that is currently under investigation. The authors recommend colonoscopy if an annual barium enema X-ray examination reveals a suspicious area, or if a rectal biopsy specimen taken through a sigmoidoscope shows epithelial dysplasia in a patient with a history of seven years or more of ulcerative colitis, if such abnormalities do not themselves result in a certain recommendation for colectomy. Severe dysplasia in a rectal biopsy specimen in a patient with long-standing ulcerative colitis is probably sufficient on its own to recommend a colectomy; but mild or moderate dysplasia seen on rectal biopsy should initiate a colonoscopy with multiple biopsies to search for dysplasia along the length of the colon (e.g., every 10 cm). Even if the physician is certain in his recommendation for a colectomy, he may at times judge a colonoscopy to be appropriate in order to impress upon his patient (or upon a surgical colleague) that the dysplasia is extensive.

The *debatable* point is thus whether a routine colonoscopy is justified when the rectal biopsy and barium enema X-ray findings are normal. The evidence seems to indicate a very small increment of benefit in performing colonoscopy under those circumstances—with risk:benefit and cost:benefit ratios probably insufficient to recommend this approach.

Patients with pseudopolyposis do not seem to be at an increased risk of the development of carcinoma simply because of the presence of pseudopolyps. Colonoscopy in such patients is sometimes difficult because of obstruction to the colonoscope if the pseudopolyps are dense. Two or three pseudopolyps should be taken for biopsy in any colonoscopic (or sigmoidoscopic) examination. If there are more than 2 or 3 pseudopolyps, one has to be selective in choosing which to take for biopsy. Any pseudopolyp that appears atypical should be subjected to biopsy in the search for carcinoma.

The other indication for colonoscopy in ulcerative colitis is in the unusual patient in whom the colitis is suspected of being active beyond the 30-cm reach of the sigmoidoscope, who has rectal sparing, and who has had a barium enema X-ray study that is inconclusive.

The appearances of the mucosa at colonoscopy are the same as those at sigmoidoscopy. The introduction of a small amount of air or carbon dioxide to distend the bowel allows a better examination.

Diseases of the colon that often spare the rectum (e.g., Crohn's disease, amebiasis, or ischemic colitis) can be diagnosed and biopsies taken at colonoscopy. When the pattern of distribution of an alternative form of colitis is an important feature, colonoscopy may be especially valuable (see Chapters 4 and 9).

FIBEROPTIC SIGMOIDOSCOPY

There has recently been introduced a fiberoptic sigmoidoscope 60 cm in length. This instrument is identical to the longer colonoscope, except that its wider diameter allows two operating channels instead of one, which may be useful on occasion (56). The fiberoptic sigmoidoscope appears to offer advantages over rigid sigmoidoscopy (though less in the management of ulcerative colitis than in the detection of occult rectal bleeding); but the situations in which fiberoptic sigmoidoscopy might be appropriate could just as easily be met with a standard long colonoscope. The term "fiberoptic sigmoidoscopy" could be used to include examinations to a depth of 60 cm with either the new flexible sigmoidoscope or the standard colonoscope. Fiberoptic sigmoidoscopy permits a more extensive examination than rigid sigmoidoscopy in most cases. However, it seems that examinations with the fiberoptic instruments are not, overall, noticeably less painful than with the rigid instrument, for a comparable examination, although there are patients who do prefer the flexible instrument for a sigmoidoscopy.

The cost of a fiberoptic sigmoidoscope is almost as high as that of a long colonoscope, which means that fiberoptic sigmoidoscopy is a considerably more expensive procedure than rigid sigmoidoscopy. In comparing fiberoptic sigmoidoscopy using the 60-cm instrument and using the standard colonoscope, the disadvantage of the 60-cm instrument is that one does not have the option of proceeding beyond a depth of 60 cm should that be judged to be necessary during the examination. Advantages of the 60-cm flexible sigmoidoscope are that it is stiffer than full-length colonoscopes, which may make the examinations easier to perform, and that it is probably sturdier than a long colonoscope and less easily damaged when less experienced operators are using it; a large institution may therefore find it useful to have a 60-cm sigmoidoscope, to save on the wear of its colonoscopes.

BIOPSY

The use of rectal biopsy in the diagnosis of ulcerative colitis is a little controversial. In general, sigmoidoscopy without biopsy should be adequate for the follow-up of the patient with diagnosed ulcerative colitis in whom the severity of the disease is to be assessed.

Once friability of the mucosa or a more severe abnormality has been observed on sigmoidoscopy, a biopsy is not necessary if the appearances are typical of ulcerative colitis. Similarly, a biopsy is not required for the normal rectum without edema or erythema, unless there is a history of bloody diarrhea on a previous occasion. A normal rectal biopsy specimen always contains a few inflammatory cells, so that an inexperienced pathologist presented with such a specimen often decides in favor of the clinician's queries about inflammation and sends a report: "Compatible with mild proctitis."

Indications

The rectal biopsy is useful in ulcerative colitis and should be performed in the following situations:

1. When sigmoidoscopic appearances are not entirely normal but are not diagnostic of ulcerative colitis. There may only be hyperemia or the absence of the normal vascular pattern. The biopsy specimen can show diagnostic changes of active or previous ulcerative colitis.
2. When the sigmoidoscopic appearances are normal but results of the barium enema X-ray examination are suggestive of ulcerative colitis.

3. When both sigmoidoscopic and barium enema X-ray findings are normal but there is a suspicion that the patient previously suffered an attack of ulcerative colitis. Even if the examining physician does not suspect ulcerative colitis, the patient may have been told by another physician that he has suffered from ulcerative colitis, and it is then useful to be able to exclude that diagnosis by means of biopsy.

4. In the exclusion of other forms of colitis. Crohn's disease of the colon, membranous colitis, amebic colitis, and bacillary dysentery are examples of conditions in which the sigmoidoscopic appearances can resemble those of ulcerative colitis. A fuller list of alternative forms of colitis and their pathology is contained in Chapter 4.

5. As a reference for the treatment of future attacks, even if there seems no doubt about the diagnosis on sigmoidoscopy. It is always possible that the patient will be under the care of another physician at the time of a subsequent attack; and it is useful for a reference biopsy to be available at that time. Reports of sigmoidoscopic appearances are very subjective, and many gastroenterologists do not generally accept without question the reports of sigmoidoscopies performed by physicians they do not know. This is a justifiable attitude; for example, one does not always know the experience of the other physician and whether or not an irritant sigmoidoscopy preparation was ordered. On the other hand, a biopsy slide (not just the pathologist's report of the biopsy) is a piece of objective evidence that should always be available for examination.

6. In the search for early carcinoma in patients with long-standing ulcerative colitis.

There may be other circumstances in which the physician will feel that scrutiny of a biopsy specimen will assist in the evaluation of the patient with ulcerative colitis; but the biopsy should always be performed for a definite reason, not simply because of a routine.

Rectal biopsy can be considered quite a safe procedure (though not entirely safe), and it is justifiable to ask patients for permission to take biopsies during the controlled evaluation of forms of drug therapy for ulcerative colitis in order to achieve an objective assessment of the response to such therapy.

Technique

Special biopsy forceps are used. These forceps are inserted through the sigmoidoscope; they have at their distal end sharp cupped blades 2 to 3 mm in diameter and are operated by a scissors mechanism at their proximal end. The forceps are inserted through the sigmoidoscope and are opened just proximal to the mucosa to be removed. The opened cupped blades are pressed gently onto the mucosa, then they are closed and the tissue is avulsed with a rotation of the wrist. A small amount of bleeding occurs from the site of biopsy. Pressure on this site with a small piece of cotton gauze held in forceps (not the biopsy forceps, because this tends to blunt the blades for future use), or with a long "Q-tip," nearly always arrests the bleeding. Sometimes the pressure may have to be applied continuously for 2 to 3 minutes (this seems a long time to the operator and the patient).

It has been stated that the safest site for biopsy is one of the rectal valves. However, more typical histology, without the excessive amounts of muscularis mucosae that are sometimes found in the valves, is obtained when the specimen is taken from flat mucosa away from the valves.

One of the dangers in performing a rectal biopsy is perforation of the bowel. Extraperitoneal perforation is less dangerous than intraperitoneal perforation; so the biopsy specimen is best taken below the peritoneal reflection, say at 10 cm from the anal margin on the posterior wall. In case a localized lesion is found in the biopsy tissue, the site of biopsy should always be recorded. If the colitis appears limited on sigmoidoscopy, i.e., it is a proctitis, biopsy specimens should be taken both from a typically involved area in the rectum and from an apparently uninvolved area, as far as possible from the inflamed rectum. When there appears to be frank ulceration, biopsy specimens should be taken from the ulcerated area and also from a nonulcerated area—the ulcerated area may have lost all its epithelium, but it is the appearances of the epithelium that are the most important for diagnosis.

Orientation

The rectal biopsy specimen should be oriented flat on a piece of filter paper, with the mucosal surface uppermost. The pathologist can give a more meaningful interpretation of a properly oriented specimen sectioned with the crypts vertical than if he receives the specimen rolled up and his technician then cuts it transversely across the crypts.

Risks and Precautions

The two risks inherent in rectal biopsy are perforation and hemorrhage. There is a risk of perforation during sigmoidoscopy without biopsy. It is the author's experience that with the biopsy forceps there is in fact less risk of perforating a mucosa that is inflamed or involved in even minimally active ulcerative colitis than of perforating normal rectal mucosa. This is probably because the presence of submucosal edema in colitis allows easier avulsion of mucosal tissue. A small perforation usually heals after a few days of bowel rest with intravenous alimentation, especially if the perforation is extraperitoneal. With peritoneal perforations that become contaminated with stool, and sometimes also with extraperitoneal perforations, the patient may need a temporary diverting colostomy. It is thus fortunate that such a complication as perforation is unusual during active ulcerative colitis, because the creation of a colostomy would be hazardous in such a situation.

The risk of hemorrhage can be minimized by avoiding rectal biopsy in patients with known disorders of clotting mechanisms and patients taking anticoagulant medications. In fact, the prothrombin time and the plasma thromboplastin time should always be checked prior to rectal biopsy. If the hemorrhage does not cease within two or three minutes of pressure on the biopsy site with cotton gauze, the next step is to insert six or eight small pieces of gauze (the number should be recorded) into the rectum; the patient should then sit still on a firm chair for an hour. The sigmoidoscopy is then repeated, and the pieces of gauze are removed. Generally this is sufficient to arrest the bleeding; but if hemorrhage is still occurring, the patient should be hospitalized and kept on intravenous fluids without oral feeding, with frequent observations of pulse and blood pressure. Transfusion may be necessary. It is extremely unusual for the bleeding to continue for longer than 24 hours. In such circumstances, a hematologist should be consulted and asked to seek and treat any disorders of the coagulation mechanisms.

Interpretation

The interpretation of the pathology of the rectal and colonic mucosa in definite or suspected ulcerative colitis has been discussed in Chapter 4.

Colonoscopic Biopsies

Colonoscopic biopsy specimens are much smaller than rectal biopsy specimens and more difficult to orient and to interpret. The indications for colonoscopic biopsy are really the same as those for rectal biopsy; it will be recalled that the indication for colonoscopy in ulcerative colitis is very often for biopsy of a suspicious localized area. Because of the smallness of the specimens, perforation and significant hemorrhage are very rare following colonoscopic biopsy, so that multiple biopsies—even up to 20 biopsies in a single examination—carry virtually no risks beyond those of the colonoscopy itself.

EXFOLIATIVE CYTOLOGY

Cytological examination of cells obtained by brushing an area suspected of being malignant can occasionally result in the diagnosis of cancer being made when biopsy specimens are normal or borderline. At every sigmoidoscopic and colonoscopic examination, a nylon cytology brush should be available for brushing lesions. All sides of the brush are rubbed onto clear glass slides, making three smears each of two or three brushings of each area. The slides are fixed immediately in ethyl alcohol.

Saline lavage of the colon has also been used as a method of obtaining cells in the search for carcinoma complicating ulcerative colitis, although it is not a widely used routine.

A specialist in cytology should interpret the cells. The Papanicolaou stain is generally used.

For details of cytological technique and interpretation, the reader should consult an appropriate text (57).

12 RADIOLOGY

Although the diagnosis of ulcerative colitis is usually made from the patient's history and sigmoidoscopic examination, it is important to delineate the extent of the disease. This can only be done by barium enema X-ray examination or by colonoscopy. The barium enema X-ray examination is easier to perform and is faster and less difficult for the patient than a colonoscopy. The place of colonoscopy was discussed in Chapter 11.

Colonoscopic studies have shown that ulcerative colitis may be more extensive than is revealed by the barium enema X-ray examination. The better the quality of the barium enema X-ray examination, the more reliable it will be in defining the extent of the ulcerative colitis. Although colonoscopically evident disease may be present in areas appearing normal in high-quality barium enema X-ray studies, the degree of inflammation in such areas can be assumed to be only mild or mild-to-moderate.

THE PLAIN ABDOMINAL X-RAY FILM

The patient with severe or fulminant ulcerative colitis is usually too ill to undergo a routine or even a modified barium enema X-ray examination; this may make the acute episode worse, or initiate a toxic megacolon or even a rupture of the colon. For such a patient, the plain abdominal X-ray film is most important; careful attention to detail will provide a great deal of information.

Air within the lumen of the colon can act as a contrast material. Since the colon is a storage organ, most patients do have some air in the colon, although a patient with severe diarrhea will usually clear the air rapidly. The normal mucosa presents a smooth interface with the retained air in the lumen. As the mucosal surface becomes eroded with the large ulcerations of severe ulcerative colitis, an irregular interface becomes apparent, particularly when contrasted on serial films (Figure 12–1). Normally, retained fecal material would interfere with such an "air-contrast" study, but this is not the case in severe ulcerative colitis in which the patient does not have formed stools.

The serosal fat layer is rarely perceived in plain X-ray films of the abdomen, since the normal bowel wall is relatively thin. In the patient with severe ulcerative colitis, thickening of the mucosa and the submucosa may develop, and this can be detected by examination of the surface of the bowel and the thin radiolucent strip on the outside of the colon.

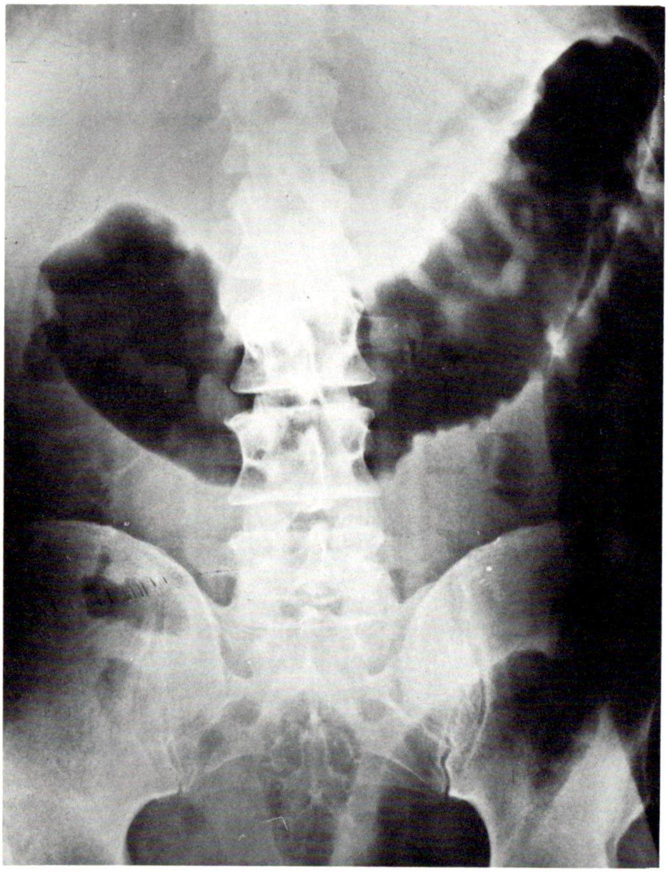

FIGURE 12–1
Plain X-ray of the abdomen demonstrating toxic dilatation of the colon complicating ulcerative colitis. Note the mucosal islands as filling defects in the air-filled, dilated transverse colon. The sigmoid colon is also dilated (*lower left*).

The plain abdominal X-ray film can also be used to screen for the presence of ankylosing spondylitis and sacroiliitis (see below, this chapter).

Acute Dilatation

Toxic megacolon affords an excellent opportunity for application of the above principles. The loss of tonicity and motility of the colon is conducive to significant air-trapping within the colonic lumen, so that the mucosal surface can be readily visualized (Figure 12–1) and an estimation can be made of the mucosal thickness, using the serosal fat line. Repeated studies are obtained with ease and allow serial comparisons during the acute episode.

The diagnosis of toxic megacolon is made on both clinical and radiological grounds. The clinical picture of the patient is as important as the radiological evidence of dilatation (Chapter 7). Some patients with long-standing ulcerative colitis may develop a chronically dilated colon that looks very similar on X-ray film to a typical toxic megacolon; however, the patient is well, with good bowel sounds and no fever, and such a condition cannot be taken to be a toxic megacolon. On the other hand, an *occult* toxic megacolon may be revealed on the X-ray film of a patient receiving large doses of steroids who may look deceptively well. In the patient who clinically fits the picture of toxic megacolon as described in Chapter 7, serial abdominal films are most important, both to follow the course of the acute episode and to determine if free perforation has occurred.

Dilatation of the colon in patients with fulminant ulcerative colitis seems to involve most often the ascending and transverse portions of the colon. Initially, only the transverse colon is seen to be dilated, probably because it possesses a mesentery, in contrast to the fixation of the ascending and descending portions of the colon. The sigmoid and descending colon normally are narrower than the rest of the colon because the bands of circular muscle are thicker and closer together (hence responsible for the occurrence of diverticular disease in the sigmoid colon).

Measurement of the largest diameter of the colon in toxic megacolon is useful, although a clinical decision should not be based solely on this parameter. Various values have been given as the point of diagnosing toxic megacolon, ranging from 10 to 13 cm. This is only one factor in the diagnosis of toxic megacolon. Perforation of the colon has occurred in some patients before this diameter was reached.

An early sign that has been noted in toxic megacolon is gaseous dilatation of part of the small intestine, probably representing a reflex paralytic ileus.

Perforation

Perforation of the colon is one of the most dreaded complications in ulcerative colitis, as described in Chapter 7. Since the patient with severe ulcerative colitis is usually receiving corticosteroid therapy, the perforation may be somewhat masked and may only be discovered on a plain abdominal X-ray film by the presence of air under one or both of the diaphragms. Thus, not only are serial films important in evaluating the acutely ill patient but upright films are mandatory. For an adequate examination, the entire diaphragm must be seen on the films. Often a single posterior-anterior chest X-ray film serves this purpose, but if the diaphragms are not well seen, the physician must be firm in his request that another set of films be taken. Free peritoneal air also may be seen in other views of the abdomen, such as in a decubitus film in an extremely debilitated patient or, when air is present in large quantities, even in the supine view.

THE BARIUM ENEMA X-RAY EXAMINATION

Ulcerative colitis is usually diagnosed from the patient's history and the sigmoidoscopic examination. Not infrequently, however, it is the barium enema X-ray study that leads to the diagnosis. This can happen when an inexperienced sigmoidoscopist reports a normal appearance of the rectal mucosa but the findings of the barium enema X-ray examination subsequently requested prove to be abnormal. It can also happen when a patient with chronic, inactive ulcerative colitis has a sigmoidoscopy that appears within normal limits (even to an experienced observer) but the barium enema X-ray film shows features indicating chronic ulcerative colitis (see below). It can happen too when the clinician feels fairly confident from the reports of other physicians that the patient has or has not got ulcerative colitis but the barium enema X-ray study is scheduled before the sigmoidoscopy for a reason of convenience.

Every patient in whom ulcerative colitis is diagnosed by sigmoidoscopy or is strongly suspected from the clinical history (despite an apparently normal sigmoidoscopy) should have a barium enema X-ray examination. If the colitis is active and firmly diagnosed on sigmoidoscopy and if immediate therapeutic decisions can be made without the information to be derived from the barium enema X-ray study, this study should be delayed until there is improvement in the severity of the colitis.

In fulminant disease, a barium enema X-ray examination might be quite dangerous; therefore, it should not be performed without due deliberation in every case. The reasons for obtaining a barium enema X-ray study are to determine the extent of disease and to detect the presence of neoplasms or of other colonic complications such as strictures.

Repeated Examinations

Occasionally, serial barium enema X-ray examinations are performed to assess the results of therapy, although this practice must be looked upon with disfavor as a general principle both because of the risk of precipitating a flare-up in quiescent disease and because of a concern about the effects of radiation exposure, particularly on the genitalia (and also because the physician should be treating the patient rather than an X-ray film).

When a patient has already had an adequate examination, a further barium enema X-ray study can be indicated for the following reasons: 1) to confirm the suspicion of a considerable increase in the extent of the disease (this indication cannot logically apply to patients already known to have total involvement of the colon with ulcerative colitis); 2) to investigate a suspicion that the patient is really suffering from Crohn's disease (although colonoscopy with multiple biopsies is more definitive in these circumstances); 3) to investigate a suspicion of a pericolic abscess or a benign stricture; and 4) to exclude the possibility of a carcinoma in any patient with ulcerative colitis who has had the disease (or any symptoms that could have been ascribed to ulcerative colitis) for more than five years. Annual barium enema X-ray examinations for the detection of carcinoma are justifiable (and recommended by the authors) in patients who have had colitis for more than seven years; but such a routine study should not be performed in an active phase of disease unless it is suspected that the symptoms indicating activity could turn out to be those of a tumor.

Preparation

Nowhere in gastroenterology does the physician's plan for preparation of the bowel prior to examination deserve more thought than in ulcerative colitis.

Overzealous cleaning of the colon can result in the flare-up of previously quiescent colitis; it can precipitate toxic megacolon in an acutely ill patient. On the other hand, poor and inadequate preparation may produce false positive findings due to residual stool; or, more commonly, poor preparation results in a worthless study that requires repetition.

A "routine" preparation should not be ordered without first assessing the patient clinically. There should be understanding and trust between physician and radiologist on this point. The patient with ulcerative colitis in remission or with mild-to-moderate disease can probably undergo the same preparation as patients without colonic disease. This preparation may range from administering a simple laxative, such as 2 oz of castor oil or phosphosoda, to a more elaborate routine involving a clear liquid diet, a potent cathartic, and a saline purgative, such as magnesium citrate, plus a suppository or a small enema. The latter routine seems to be better in several respects; the patient tolerates it better and lacks severe dehydration, and the improved quality of colonic cleaning makes it possible to obtain good film. Since the barium enema X-ray examination is looked upon by the patient as a major chore, all efforts should be made to obtain a good study with the first examination.

Recently, the technique of saline lavage without laxatives or enemas has been described, using large amounts of a physiological saline (including potassium) taken orally (58); this preparation is suitable in inactive or mild-to-moderate ulcerative colitis, although it is unsuitable for patients with cardiac or renal disease.

It is well to remember that retained stool clinging to the mucosa may resemble the pseudopolyps and gross ulcerations of more severe ulcerative colitis. Thus, every effort should be made to make the bowel as free from fecal material as possible prior to examination.

Performance of a sigmoidoscopy and a barium enema X-ray examination on the same day should be avoided. Although, on first thought, it would seem to be a kindness to the patient not to have to undergo two preparations and make two visits to the hospital, several factors argue against this. As discussed in the preceding chapter, most sigmoidoscopies in patients with proved or suspected ulcerative colitis should be unprepared; so this examination can be performed at any time. A sigmoidoscopy, no matter how carefully performed, even without the deliberate addition of air, always allows considerable amounts of air to enter the colon; and when sigmoidoscopy is performed just before a barium enema X-ray examination, the air introduced often gets pushed into the cecum by the barium. If the ileocecal valve is patent, the cecal air either will not allow adequate visualization of the cecum with barium or will cause pain as the radiologist attempts to add more barium.

Certainly, if a rectal biopsy is performed, barium should not be introduced for at least another five days, since the pressure of the enema on a weakened bowel wall has been known to lead to perforation (59).

In the more severe cases of ulcerative colitis, the preparation must be modified to suit the clinical condition of the patient. Some or all of the laxatives may be omitted, with only tapwater or saline enemas administered (although, unfortunately, the latter often do not effectively clean the ascending or even the transverse colon). However, diarrhea itself is a fairly effective purgative. For the patient with severe ulcerative colitis who is considered able to tolerate instillation of barium, a clear liquid diet often is required for at least one day before the examination. This is less than satisfactory in some patients, since even semi-formed fecal material may cling to the mucosa and give a false impression regarding the extent and severity of disease. In patients of this type, perhaps the saline lavage described above may find its useful place.

Technique

A barium enema X-ray examination in a patient with ulcerative colitis requires more care than may be customary in a routine examination; therefore, the radiologist should always have information about the patient's clinical condition and must feel free to question the patient's physician if there is a possibility that the patient is too ill to undergo the examination. Certainly, the radiologist does not want to be instrumental in precipitating a toxic megacolon or perforation of the bowel.

Many patients with ulcerative colitis have a fear of barium enema X-ray examinations because of pain during the procedure, panic about not being able to hold the barium (with consequent soiling and embarrassment), and sometimes the recollection of having had a flare-up of colitis after a previous examination. The patient must be convinced by the physician of the importance of that particular examination.

A rectal balloon should be used with caution, particularly if the rectal mucosa is severely inflamed.

Glucagon, 1 to 2 mg, may be injected intramuscularly to provide temporary paralysis of the colon, relieving both the discomfort secondary to spasm and the fear of losing the barium. This agent can be used without concern in the diabetic patient, although it should be avoided in an acutely ill patient who might develop a toxic megacolon.

In the severely ill patient with fever and with irregularity of the mucosal outline as seen on plain abdominal X-ray films, serious consideration should be given to avoiding the barium enema X-ray examination altogether; for the boggy, edematous mucosa can be easily perforated. Naturally, in such a patient, an experienced radiologist must be present for every moment of the examination, and there should be slow and cautious instillation of barium. The practice of allowing a technician to fill the colon prior to the radiologist's entrance on the scene is not suitable if ulcerative colitis is suspected, and the practice is actually dangerous in the presence of moderate or severe ulcerative colitis.

Tannic acid should not be added to the barium mixture when performing a barium enema X-ray examination on a patient with ulcerative colitis. This additive, which gives superb mucosal views on postevacuation or air-contrast studies, has been responsible for several deaths in patients with ulcerative colitis because the tannic acid was absorbed through the inflamed mucosa and produced hepatic necrosis (60).

The performance of the barium enema X-ray examination can be accomplished with a minimum of movement on the part of the severely ill, debilitated patient. A lateral view of the rectum and good postevacuation films are important, as discussed below. All or most of the barium can be drained from the colon while the patient is still on the examining table, so that a rush to the toilet afterwards should be unnecessary.

APPEARANCES ON BARIUM ENEMA X-RAY EXAMINATION

Retrorectal (Presacral) Space

Long-standing inflammation produces mucosal and submucosal thickening in some but not all patients with ulcerative proctitis or ulcerative colitis. This is seen in the lateral view of the barium-filled rectum as an increase in the distance between the posterior rectal wall and the anterior surface of the sacrum, which should be less than one centimeter. An increase of this space of between 1 and 2 cm is suggestive of long-standing disease, and over 2 cm is considered definite evidence for submucosal thickening (Figure 12–2). The rectal mucosa itself may

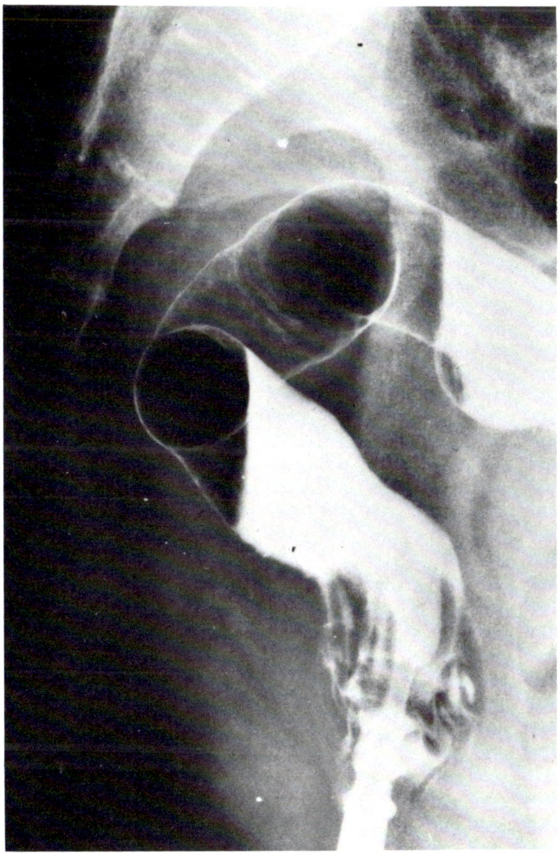

FIGURE 12–2
Lateral X-ray view of barium-filled rectum in ulcerative colitis, showing a retrorectal, presacral space.

be irregular due to ulceration, but frequently it appears normal, in parallel to a relative rectal sparing effect, as seen on sigmoidoscopy, which can occur even in severe ulcerative colitis.

Filled Views

When ulceration becomes severe, irregularity of the mucosal-barium interface becomes obvious. Radiological evidence of ulcerations of the colon can range from simple serration of the mucosa to large "collar-button" ulcers (Figures 12–3 and 12–4).

Serration

Serration of the colonic mucosa is produced by the barium filling tiny ulcerations. This change may be seen only in the distal sigmoid, or it can spread proximally to involve the entire colon, depending upon the acuteness and

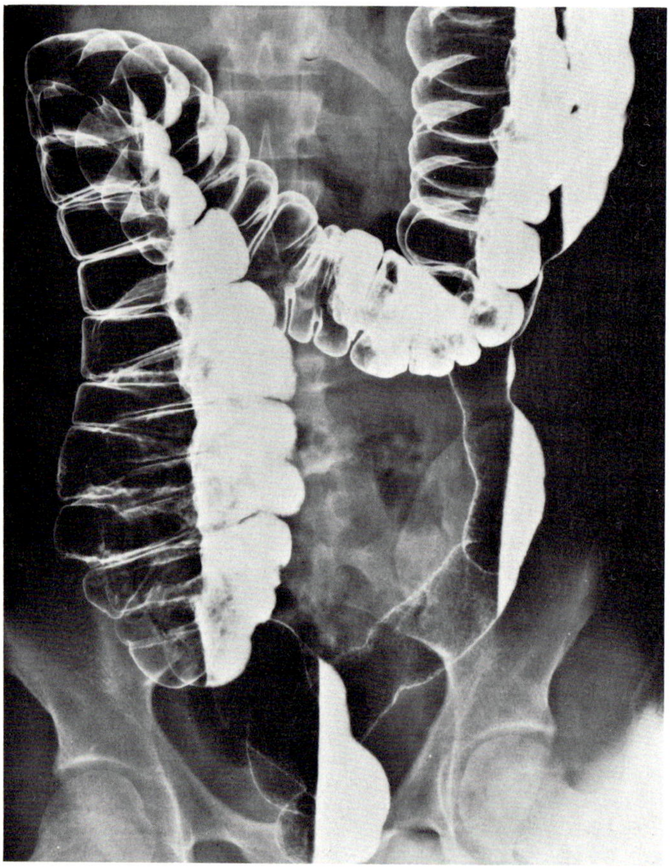

FIGURE 12–3
Barium enema X-ray in a patient with ulcerative colitis involving the descending and sigmoid colon and the rectum. The haustra are absent in the affected segment of the colon.

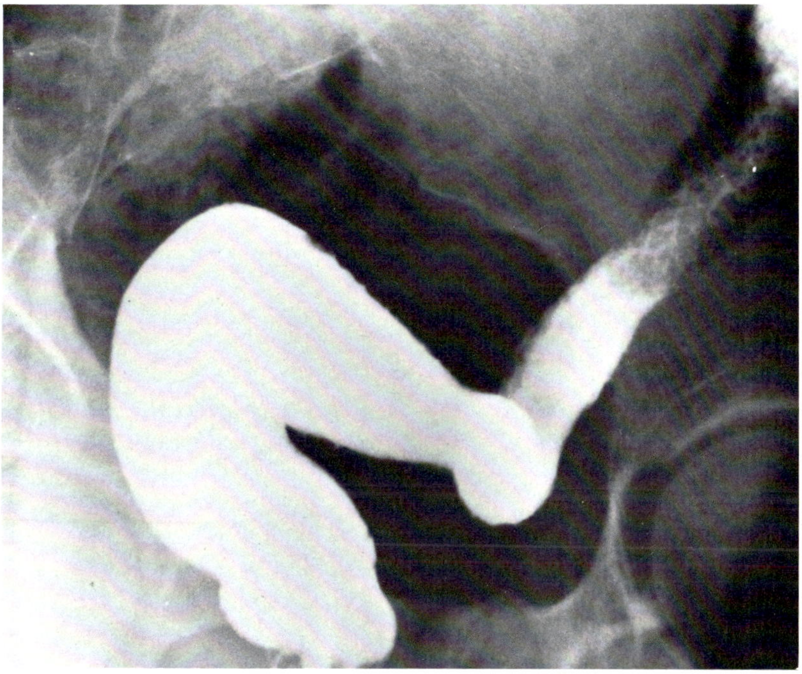

FIGURE 12–4
Barium enema X-ray of the rectum and sigmoid in a patient with ulcerative colitis. Note the serrated, ulcerated mucosa.

severity of the attack. Usually the serrations are seen to involve the bowel wall circumferentially at whatever level they are seen. It is this degree of ulceration that is observed in the terminal ileum in so-called "backwash ileitis," representing superficial mucosal ulcers in a slightly dilated ileum, in contrast to the deeper fissures and narrowing of Crohn's disease (see Figure 12–9).

Large supine and prone films often are better than small spot films for detecting small ulcerations of the mucosa; this is due to technical factors, better resolution being obtained when the X-ray tube is farther away from the film. Spot films are useful for examining the flexures and the sigmoid in various oblique views to look for intraluminal filling defects, but the large 11 × 14 in (28 × 35 cm) films provide more information about the status and extent of the ulcerative colitis.

Large Ulcers

Larger ulcers usually correlate with more extensive involvement in the more acutely ill patient who has severe diarrhea and often weight loss as well as rectal bleeding. Deeper ulcers often appear to widen as they burrow into the submucosa, creating the "collar-button" ulcers of severe ulcerative colitis. These ulcers are also seen in severe amebiasis; but with the decline in the incidence of that disease they are more commonly found in ulcerative colitis. The "collar-button" ulcers of ulcerative colitis often involve the colon circumferentially, in contrast to the deep ulceration of Crohn's colitis. The deep fissures of Crohn's colitis may resemble these ulcers but usually are narrower and more irregular in their spacing. Not infrequently, the radiologist cannot distinguish between these two types of inflammatory bowel disease when severe ulceration is present, particularly if one segment of the colon is more affected than another.

As the disease becomes more severe and the ulcers become larger in area, loss of the colonic mucosal surface occurs in some places and healing occurs with excessive mucosal regeneration. The mucosa now appears to support intraluminal filling defects, the so-called pseudopolyps; or the colon can be literally carpeted with them (Figure 12–5).

Foreshortened Colon

The acute inflammation of ulcerative colitis also may affect the muscularis mucosae and even the muscularis propria, producing a smooth ahaustral,

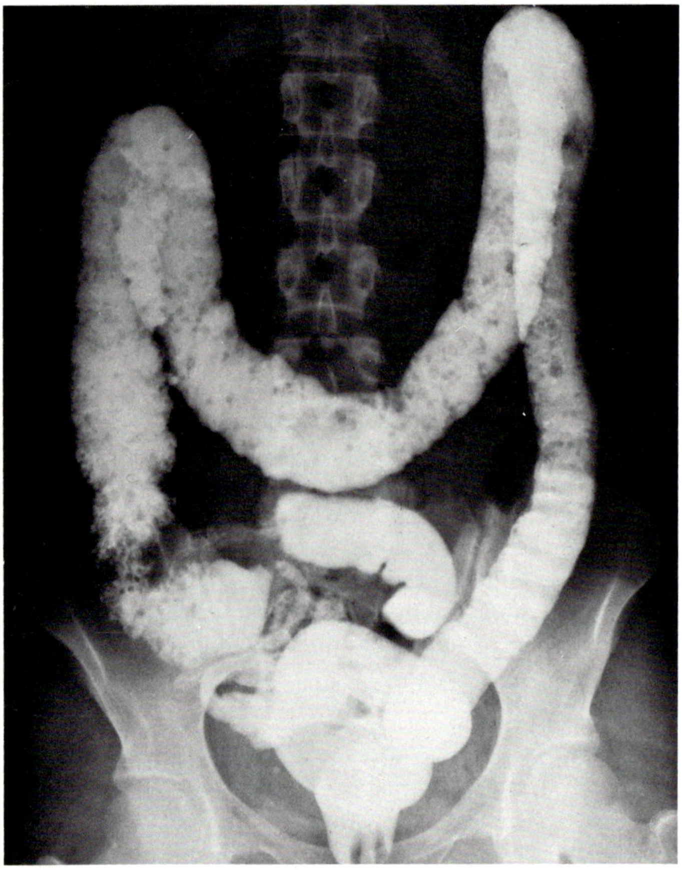

FIGURE 12–5
Barium enema X-ray in a patient with ulcerative colitis involving the whole colon, showing extensive pseudopolyposis of the ascending, transverse, and descending colon.

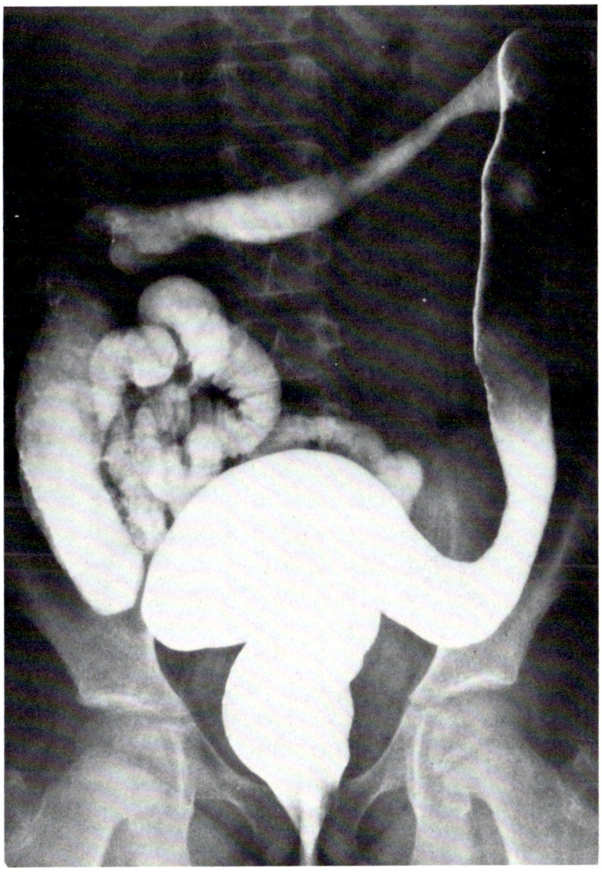

FIGURE 12–6
Barium enema X-ray in a patient with chronic ulcerative colitis causing foreshortening of the colon and benign strictures at the hepatic flexure and in the left transverse colon.

frequently foreshortened, colon (Figure 12–6). These changes are potentially reversible during a first attack of colitis when the shortening represents spasm and edema, rather than chronic muscular hypertrophy. If the colon has not become shrunken in length and width, there is a good chance that reversal is possible.

Since a correlation appears to exist between the extent of disease and the prognosis, the radiologist should comment on the most proximal extent of disease, for example, thus: "Inflammation involving the hepatic flexure with the ascending colon appearing to be normal."

Postevacuation Films

A great deal of information can be obtained about subtle mucosal ulcerations by scrutinizing the postevacuation film. Tiny ulcers are often masked by the barium itself on the filled views of the colon and can be seen best after much of the barium has been evacuated. A fine granularity of the mucosa seen on postevacuation films may be the only radiological sign of ulcerative colitis. What appears to be normal on filled films may be seen as extensive ulcerative colitis on good postevacuation views of the mucosa. The postevacuation film should always be considered in determining the extent of disease, for it may show much more serious and extensive longitudinal involvement than is initially apparent. In a small series of patients with normal filled views but extensive ulceration on the postevacuation films, the prognosis was the same as that of extensive ulcerative colitis (61).

Chronic Changes

Long-standing ulcerative colitis produces chronic, irreversible changes in the muscularis as well as the mucosa of the colon. Although considered a mucosal disease, ulcerative colitis causes the muscularis to become thickened. This results in a decrease in both the width and the length of the colon, creating foreshortening of the colon, with loss of the flexures and even of the sigmoid curve. Eventually, a functionless *microcolon* can result, consisting simply of a tube connecting the ileum to the anus.

Pseudopolyposis

Pseudopolyps are considered to be a manifestation of chronic change, although they have been known to appear following the first diagnosed attack of ulcerative colitis. They appear as round filling defects in the barium-filled lumen (Figure 12–5). Although considered a sign of more severe ulcerative colitis, the presence of pseudopolyps gives no information about the present state of the patient with regard to the activity of the disease. There does not seem to be any correlation between pseudopolyposis and carcinoma in that pseudopolyps themselves do not become malignant. However, the same general rule about long-standing extensive disease in ulcerative colitis would apply to the patient with chronic disease and pseudopolyposis extending throughout the colon.

Strictures

Morphological features distinguishing benign from malignant strictures in ulcerative colitis were described in Chapter 7. These characteristics are best appreciated radiologically (see Figures 12–6 and 12–8).

THE AIR-CONTRAST BARIUM ENEMA X-RAY EXAMINATION (Figure 12–7)

Usually, the regular single-contrast barium enema X-ray examination provides sufficient information about the severity and extent of ulcerative colitis, so that there is no need to resort to the more time-consuming, complex, and potentially more dangerous air-contrast study. The routine use of air-contrast studies in ulcerative colitis is not to be recommended; for the patient must undergo a more stringent preparation than with the routine study so as to eliminate all fecal material from the colon, and, furthermore, the pumping of air into the bowel has been known to cause perforation.

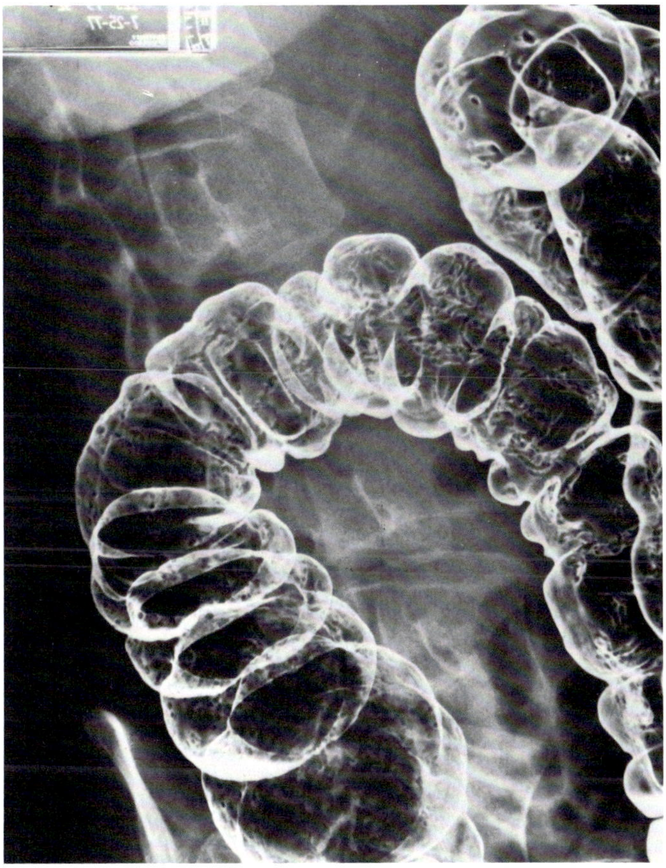

FIGURE 12–7
Air-contrast barium enema X-ray showing pseudopolyposis in a patient with inactive ulcerative colitis.

Although one might expect mucosal detail to be better with an air-contrast study, a certain amount of barium must cling to the mucosa to demonstrate the ulcerations and this quantity of barium is often enough to give the same information on the postevacuation films of a single-contrast examination.

The situation in which the air-contrast technique is of significant benefit is in the search for neoplastic change complicating long-standing ulcerative colitis (Figure 12–8); in fact, the authors recommend the use of the air-contrast technique in this situation provided that the ulcerative colitis is quiescent. Luminal filling defects, particularly when isolated, should be considered as possible carcinoma. Any area of stiffness of the mucosa or slight irregularity in an otherwise smooth segment of the colon should raise the suspicion of carcinoma. Unfortunately, even the most carefully performed studies will often miss the superficial form of mucosal carcinoma occurring secondary to ulcerative colitis. Suspicious changes found in a barium enema X-ray examination of a patient with ulcerative colitis of more than five years' duration must be followed up by means of a total colonoscopy with multiple biopsies (see Chapter 11).

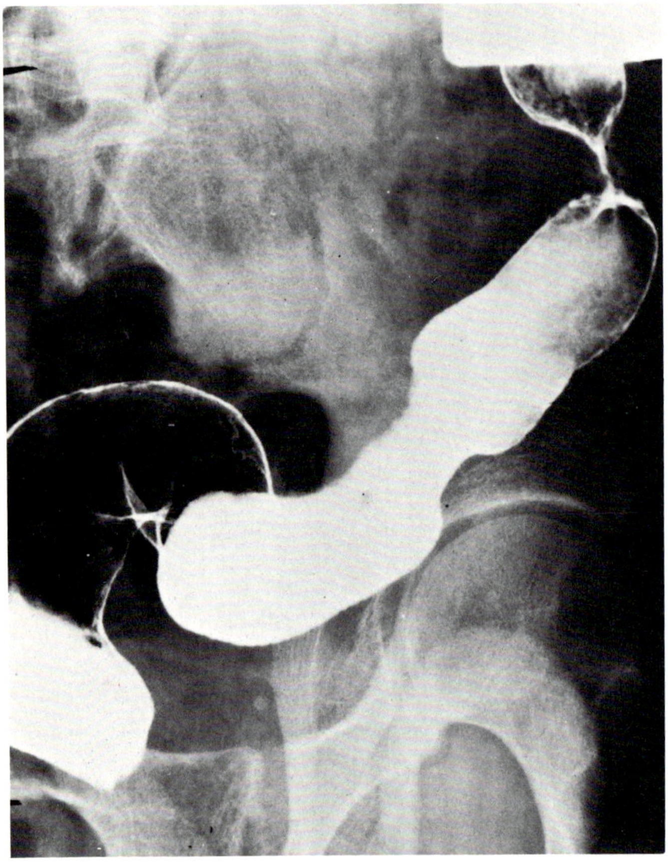

FIGURE 12–8
Barium enema X-ray of the sigmoid colon in a patient with chronic ulcerative colitis complicated by a malignant stricture *(upper right)*.

THE SMALL BOWEL FOLLOW-THROUGH X-RAY SERIES

The usefulness of the small bowel X-ray series in diagnosed ulcerative colitis is limited to the information it provides about the terminal ileum; and usually that area is better seen on the barium enema X-ray film, particularly if the ileocecal valve has been rendered incompetent by the disease. The colon should never be evaluated by an antegrade study such as the last phase of the small bowel series, for the colon has not been properly prepared and cannot be distended. A false impression of extensive colonic disease can be obtained in this fashion.

A small bowel follow-through X-ray series is an essential study if there is the slightest question that the patient may be suffering from Crohn's disease, rather than ulcerative colitis. The terminal ileum in patients with ulcerative colitis should be normal unless the entire colon is diseased. In the latter situation, the inflammation can extend proximally through the ileocecal valve into the terminal ileum. The inflammation of the terminal ileum involves only the mucosa, so that that part of the small bowel is dilated, rather than contracted, and superficial ulcerations may be present, rather than the deep fissures of Crohn's disease. Probably too much emphasis has been given to "backwash ileitis," since it is merely a reflection of total colonic involvement with ulcerative colitis.

A barium meal with a small bowel follow-through X-ray series is probably wise at some stage in the study of a patient with suspected ulcerative colitis as part of the initial evaluation of the gastrointestinal tract (see Chapter 10).

DIFFERENTIAL DIAGNOSIS

Barium X-ray studies of both the colon and the small intestine assist in differentiating ulcerative colitis from clinically similar conditions (for a discussion of these conditions, see Chapter 9). In the irritable colon syndrome the X-ray studies should be entirely normal, as they should be also in cases of rectal bleeding due solely to hemorrhoids. The localized noncolitic diseases (carcinoma, diverticulosis, polyps) have their own specific features. Laxative abuse can cause loss of haustrations and smooth narrowings of the colon (the cathartic colon), but there is no mucosal irregularity.

The "colitic" group of diseases (Chapter 9) can be divided into those that tend to produce diffuse changes in the colon and those that usually cause segmental abnormalities, with the remainder of the colon appearing normal.

Fine, diffuse mucosal changes are seen in the various acute infections of the gastrointestinal tract which involve the colon (viral gastroenteritis and infections with *Shigella, Salmonella,* and toxigenic *Escherichia coli*). There may be diffuse mucosal spiculations which (in shigellosis) may lead to more severe ulcerations. On the other hand (and more commonly), there may be no abnormalities on the barium enema X-ray film, or else the colonic mucosa just appears to have smooth but rather edematous folds; the latter appearance is most likely to be produced by a heavy, watery diarrhea and can be seen in cholera and occasionally in giardiasis, neither of which causes significant colonic inflammation.

In amebiasis, colonic ulcerations are often diffuse, though not necessarily involving the whole colon, and they are apt to be deeper than those of the more acute infections. An edematous inflammatory excrescence, known as an ameboma, may mimic a carcinoma on X-ray studies.

In membranous colitis, there may be diffuse or segmental ulcerations, which sometimes are fine ulcerations but more typically are deeper and nodular. Ischemic colitis nearly always causes segmental lengths of ulcerated colon, most commonly at the splenic flexure, and these ulcers are classically deep and "thumbprinted"; there may, however, be finer ulcerations. Ischemic colitis may heal with stricture formation.

Coarse abnormalities mostly limited to the rectum may be seen in lymphogranuloma venereum, gonorrhea, histoplasmosis, candidiasis, and anorectal tuberculosis; in leukemic and lymphomatous infiltrations; in the solitary rectal ulcer syndrome; and in Behçet's proctitis. The specific interpretation of abnormalities confined to the rectum that are seen in barium enema X-ray studies is not important, because this area can always be visualized and biopsy specimens taken on sigmoidoscopy.

Radiation proctitis can be confused with ulcerative colitis. Haustrations in the sigmoid may be lost; the bowel may appear foreshortened; and occasionally fine mucosal irregularities may be seen.

Finally, comment must be made on the radiological differentiation of Crohn's disease from ulcerative colitis. Like the endoscopic differentiation, this can be difficult. The features suggestive of a diagnosis of Crohn's disease (Figure 12–9) correspond to those described in Chapter 11 for the endoscopic differentiation of these conditions. These features divide themselves into three groups: 1) those related to the anatomical distribution of Crohn's disease—a patchy distribution with intervening normal areas of colon ("skip" lesions), abnormality of one side of a segment of the colon with the opposite mucosa appearing normal, rectal sparing, or any evidence of involvement of the small intestine (a small bowel follow-through X-ray series can be critical in making this diagnostic distinction); 2) those related to the mucosal features of Crohn's disease—deeper, fissured ulcers, more edematous mucosal folds between the

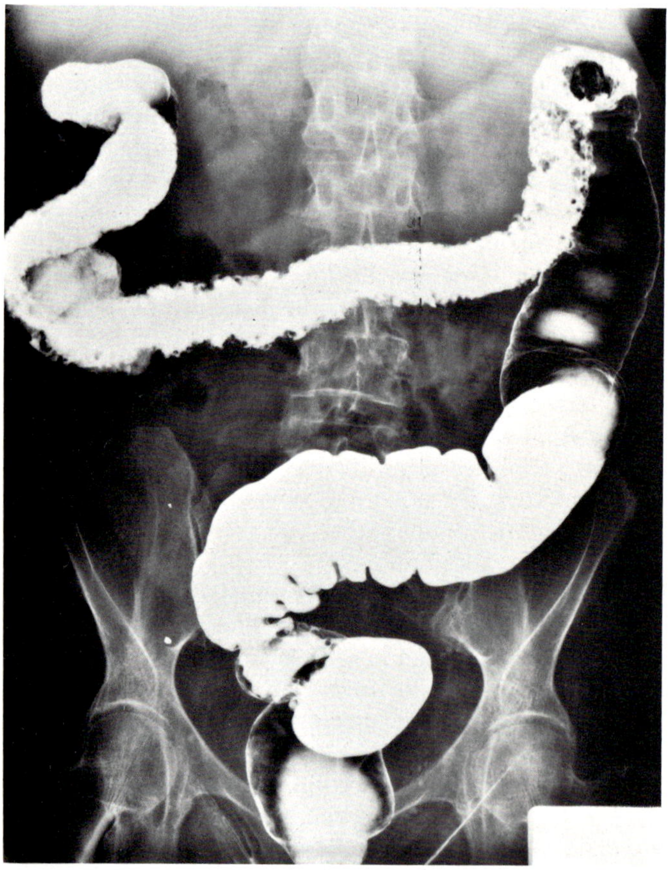

FIGURE 12–9
Barium enema X-ray in a patient with Crohn's disease involving the ascending and transverse colon. The descending colon, sigmoid, and rectum are spared.

ulcers (causing an impression of "cobblestones"); and 3) those related to specific complications of Crohn's disease—in particular, fistulas from the bowel to other abdominal organs (including other parts of the bowel) or to the skin. However, in up to 25% of cases, it may be impossible to distinguish Crohn's disease and ulcerative colitis on radiological grounds (62).

EVALUATION OF THE SYSTEMIC COMPLICATIONS

Ankylosing Spondylitis and Sacroiliitis

Ankylosing spondylitis and sacroiliitis are related complications that are diagnosed radiologically. The features may be apparent on a plain abdominal X-ray (e.g., the preliminary film of a barium enema examination); but detailed evaluation requires directed views of the thoracic and lumbosacral spine and the sacroiliac joints to be taken. In the spine, ankylosing spondylitis is characterized by a loss of the normal lumbar lordosis, together with narrowing of the intervertebral joint spaces, calcification of the cartilaginous discs and the longitudinal spinal ligaments, and osteophyte formation (Figure 12–10). Sacroiliitis appears as narrowing, blurring, and juxta-articular sclerosis of one or (usually) both sacroiliac joints.

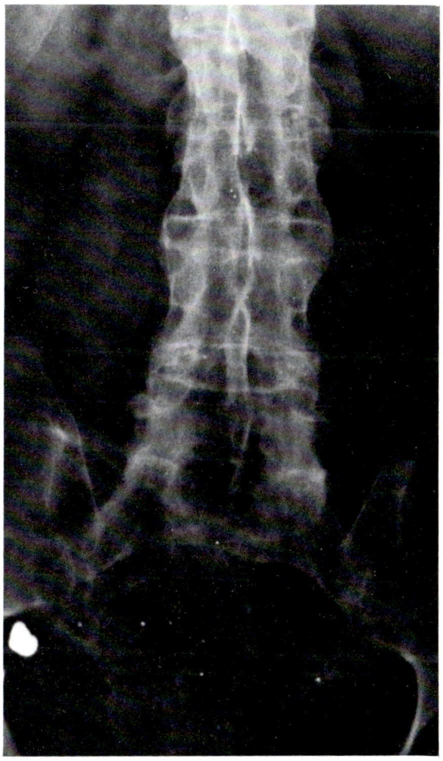

FIGURE 12–10
X-ray of the lumbosacral spine of a patient with ulcerative colitis complicated by ankylosing spondylitis. Note the calcification of the intervertebral ligaments. Note also the obliteration of the sacroiliac joints.

Other Systemic Complications

A number of the other systemic complications of ulcerative colitis require radiological investigations, e.g., intravenous pyelography for renal complications and various techniques of cholangiography for hepatobiliary complications. A plain abdominal X-ray film may demonstrate renal or ureteric calculi, or gallstones may be seen (not a specific complication of ulcerative colitis but useful in evaluating the hepatobiliary complications). The respective radiological studies for the diagnosis of the systemic complications were discussed with each complication in Chapter 8.

IV

Management

13

MEDICAL TREATMENT

MEDICAL OR SURGICAL TREATMENT?

The treatment of ulcerative colitis can be said to be primarily medical, but with the option of surgery which may become mandatory in certain situations. Surgical removal of the entire colon and rectum does completely cure the disease; however, the risks and discomforts of the operation and the necessity for a permanent ileostomy make the first choice medical rather than surgical therapy. The forms of medical treatment available can be very effective in suppressing the disease, although they have to be used with care and with consideration of their potential hazards. In general, medical treatment is used until surgery either is indicated because of a specific indication or is judged to give a better all-round outlook, taking into account both survival and quality of life.

In many instances, the decision as to whether to remove the colon is not clear-cut, and the personal views of the patient can weigh heavily on such a decision. It is the duty of the physician to judge the moment when surgery would be preferable and to ensure that the patient not only is asked for his or her reactions to the alternatives but also is fully informed as to what the alternatives would mean. Very often, the physician finds patients who would clearly benefit from surgery refusing to have an operation from a lack of appreciation of how much better they would feel and how much better their general health would be. Likewise, though less often, he finds patients requesting a surgical cure when they can be satisfactorily treated, with little risk, by medical means.

This chapter will give an account of the medical management of patients with ulcerative colitis. Chapter 16 describes the surgical therapy of the disease and lists the indications for surgical intervention. The commonest indication is "failure of medical therapy," and it is a matter of judgment when medical therapy really has failed. Toxic dilatation of the colon, although a relative indication for surgery, is in a sense a sign of failed medical therapy; initially, the condition can sometimes be treated medically, provided it is understood that surgery may be required urgently.

FORMS OF MEDICAL THERAPY

The forms of medical therapy will be dealt with separately in the following account. They can be classified as specific (treatment with drugs that suppress the disease); resuscitative (such as fluid and nutritional replacement); symptomatic (normalization of bowel habit, control of pain); and preventive (avoidance of aggravating agents).

CONSIDERATIONS IN THE USE OF MEDICAL THERAPY

The medical approach to therapy may involve one or more of the various forms of treatment. Their use is largely dictated by the degree of activity of the disease and, to a certain extent, by the history of the disease activity and the results of previous therapeutic attempts. Patients who are diagnosed as having ulcerative colitis need not necessarily be given any treatment at all if they are asymptomatic or their colitis is mild. The most convenient approach is to classify patients as having mild, moderate, or severe ulcerative colitis, or quiescent disease; the criteria for such a grading were outlined in Chapter 10. Grades of activity in between these can be designated as very mild, mild-to-moderate, and moderate-to-severe.

Patients with severe disease require hospitalization; those with mild disease usually do not. In the case of moderate disease, the decision on hospitalization can be influenced by the patient's convenience and the availability of hospital beds; ideally, hospitalization is preferable, especially in a first attack of ulcerative colitis.

CORTICOSTEROIDS AND CORTICOTROPIN

Corticosteroids and corticotropin (ACTH) are of undoubted benefit in the treatment of most patients with ulcerative colitis, at least in the short term. Corticosteroids can be used systemically (parenterally or orally) or topically in the rectum. They are effective in suppressing an attack of the disease and in inducing a remission that usually, but by no means always, persists after they are withdrawn. Their long-term use is fraught with side effects and has been shown by Truelove (63) to be ineffective in preventing relapse of quiescent disease.

Corticosteroids are preferred to ACTH because the steroids can be given orally in moderate doses, whereas ACTH always has to be given by injection; also, although Truelove (63) found that ACTH was more effective than hydrocortisone in the treatment of a relapse (but not of a first attack), the difference was not very great and there were more side effects with ACTH than with hydrocortisone treatment. Some physicians who are experienced with ACTH still prescribe it, and their practice can be justified.

Corticotropin acts via a stimulating effect on the adrenal cortex to induce the synthesis and release of endogenous hydrocortisone. Hydrocortisone and other glucocorticoids are effective in ulcerative colitis by virtue of their anti-inflammatory action. They suppress the immune response that is the basis of the lesion in ulcerative colitis (although virtually nothing is known about the antigenic stimulus to that response). Hydrocortisone has also been shown to have an effect in promoting sodium reabsorption from the colon, an effect that is known with the mineralocorticoids; and it is possible that this action plays a part in assisting the anti-inflammatory action of the steroids in producing symptomatic improvement by reducing diarrhea in patients with ulcerative colitis.

Systemic Steroids in Use

The corticosteroids currently used in ulcerative colitis are hydrocortisone, prednisone, prednisolone, and methylprednisolone. Dexamethasone, betamethasone, and triamcinolone have been used, but they do not seem to be as effective as the other steroids mentioned; triamcinolone can give rise to a proximal myopathy. Prednisone is metabolized in the liver to prednisolone; so except in patients with liver disease, who should receive prednisolone, there is no difference as to the choice between these two steroids. Some physicians prefer prednisone, some prednisolone, but one might choose prednisolone because it is the active form. In the United States prednisone is more widely used than prednisolone because of its slightly lower cost. In this discussion, the use of prednisone will be described, although prednisolone can be substituted at the same dosage. Prednisone is preferred to hydrocortisone because prednisone has less salt- and fluid-retaining mineralocorticoid activity. Methylprednisolone has even a little less mineralocorticoid activity and is being prescribed by many physicians. There seems nothing to indicate that in the choice of hydrocortisone, prednisone, or methylprednisolone there is any greater anti-inflammatory action with one than with the others when these drugs are used at biologically equivalent doses. The authors normally prescribe prednisone.

When a patient does not appear to be responding to one corticosteroid, it is often helpful to change to a different one, and a beneficial response can occur; this is an empirical finding. Another empirical observation is that a corticosteroid in use can be more effective when the patient is optimally nourished, having normal plasma albumin levels and no anemia, than when he suffers from malnutrition and anemia resulting from the colitis. If an effective dosage of steroid is being used, such as 30 mg daily of prednisone, the absence of a detectable moon-face cushingoid facies is often an indication of an ineffectual corticosteroid effect on the disease; and it may be necessary to improve the nutritional status of the patient, to correct anemia or hypoalbuminemia, to increase the dosage of the drug, or to prescribe an alternative steroid.

Side Effects

Corticosteroids have their undesirable side effects. Unfortunately, the development of these side effects more or less parallels the anti-inflammatory effectiveness of the drug with any particular dose. The physician prescribing these drugs is always compromising between giving a larger dose to increase the anti-inflammatory effect and lowering the dose to avoid side effects.

The side effects of the glucocorticoids are well known. They include the development of a moon-faced facial appearance, facial hair (with a thinning of scalp hair), truncal obesity with some wasting of the limb muscles, a posterior cervical "buffalo" hump, easy bruising, abdominal striae, and acneiform pimples—all of these having an adverse bearing on the patient's cosmetic appearance. Long-term steroid therapy can lead to subcapsular cataract formation in the eye.

The adrenal steroids can interfere with the physiology and metabolism of the steroids of sexual activity, causing menstrual irregularities in women and infertility in both sexes. Adrenal steroids have been reported to be teratogenic to the fetus, but the evidence for this is not strong. There is an impaired response of the body's cellular defense mechanisms to infection, so that infections are prone to occur (especially bacterial infections arising from the diseased bowel) and to exacerbate the patient's general illness and thence the activity of the colitis. Candidiasis and other fungal infections can develop with steroid use. In patients receiving long-term steroid therapy, there is a tendency for the development of pulmonary tuberculosis, or inactive tuberculous infection may be reactivated. The importance of this in ulcerative colitis is that ileocecal tuberculosis can mimic Crohn's disease, which itself has to be differentiated from ulcerative colitis.

Catabolic Effects

The glucocorticoids have a catabolic effect on tissue, resulting in poor healing of wounds, wasting of muscle and lymphoid tissue, and a loss of nitrogen and potassium from the body. In children, the use of steroids on a long-term basis prevents growth and delays puberty. A catabolic effect on the gastric and duodenal mucosa gives rise probably to an increased tendency to the development of peptic ulceration. In the patient who has a peptic ulcer, enteric-coated prednisone can be used if steroids continue to be required, and antacids can be given. Enteric-coated preparations have the disadvantage that the steroid may be incompletely absorbed, especially in patients with intestinal disease. The authors do not routinely use the enteric-coated drugs; nor do they recommend prophylactic antacids. The antacid preparations in use contain cations that exacerbate diarrhea, and also they frequently contain sodium which summates with the sodium-retaining effects of the steroids. Another result of the catabolic effect of the steroids is the breakdown of the bone matrix, leading to osteoporosis and resulting in fractures of the vertebrae. The glucocorticoids promote protein breakdown to glucose; and hyperglycemia and diabetes can result from their use.

Effects on Electrolyte Balance

None of the glucocorticoids in use in treating ulcerative colitis is without some mineralocorticoid effect; and salt and water retention and loss of potassium from the kidneys are side effects of the steroid drugs. Congestive cardiac failure can occur when the heart is not entirely healthy. The tendency to heart failure is exacerbated by the anemia frequently caused by ulcerative colitis. The salt retention can aggravate the tendency to edema caused by the hypoalbuminemia of the bowel disease. The hypoalbuminemia itself can be aggravated by the catabolic effects of the steroids. The potassium loss can be troublesome because the inflamed colon in ulcerative colitis is already losing excessive amounts of the potassium ion. Salt retention from prolonged use of the steroids can lead to the development of systemic hypertension. Rarely, steroids lead to ischemic lesions; those reported include pancreatitis and aseptic necrosis of the femoral heads.

Psychological Changes

The steroids can also have effects on the mood of the patient. They can lead to depression, or mania, or to a sense of euphoria; and sleeplessness can be a side effect. Patients receiving steroids have been known to commit suicide as a result of their psychosis. The patient's appetite can increase. This can be useful in nutritionally depleted patients with ulcerative colitis, but some patients become excessively obese.

False Assessments of Disease with Steroid Therapy

Some of the side effects of the steroid drugs can give rise to difficulties in assessing the severity of the disease in patients with ulcerative colitis. The most dangerous complication is silent perforation of the colon, with silent peritonitis. The peritonitis can be particularly virulent in this situation because the steroid is inhibiting the formation of fibrous tissue to limit the spread of the infection. The physician must be aware of this possible complication; but it is probably true that the steroid, used correctly, can benefit the patient with ulcerative colitis who is a candidate for perforation by suppressing the disease and preventing the perforation from occurring. Since the steroids are anti-inflammatory, they are antipyretic; however, remission of pyrexia in ulcerative colitis following the use of steroids is not necessarily an indication that the patient is recovering as rapidly as might be suggested by a fall in body temperature. Also, the patient can give an unduly optimistic account of his own symptoms, as a result of steroid-induced euphoria, which is commoner and more subtle than steroid-induced depression. On the other hand, a high total leukocyte count may give a falsely gloomy impression of the disease activity, for the steroids themselves can give rise to a polymorphonuclear leukocytosis with an accompanying lymphopenia.

Indications and Contraindications

In practice, steroids are usually absolutely indicated in treating moderate and severe ulcerative colitis, but when the harm resulting from their use would outweigh the benefit of their anti-inflammatory effects, as in mild colitis, they should be withheld if possible; surgery should be considered in the most severe attacks. When there is colonic perforation or peritonitis, surgery should be performed and steroids should only be used to maintain sufficient adrenocortical function for the body to cope with the disease and the operation. When there is a walled-off extracolonic abscess, surgery rather than steroids should be the treatment, but sometimes steroids can and should be continued. Steroids can be used in toxic dilatation of the colon provided the dilatation is not great and provided there is objective evidence of improvement in the patient's condition within a few hours of the commencement of the steroid therapy.

From the description of steroid side effects, one can deduce other contraindications to the use of steroids, although these will be relative rather than absolute. Patients who already are affected by conditions that are side effects of the steroids are, of course, especially liable to have these conditions adversely influenced by steroid use. Among these patients are those with infections, with peptic ulcers, skeletal demineralization, diabetes mellitus, cardiac disease, and hypertension, and patients with a history of psychiatric disturbance.

Suppression of the Adrenal Cortex

The administration of exogenous adrenal glucocorticoids has an inhibitory effect on the hypothalamo-pituitary-adrenal axis. The steroids inhibit the hypothalamic release of corticotropin-releasing hormone (CRH), thereby diminishing the output of ACTH. This results in a lack of hormone synthesis by the adrenal cortex, which becomes atrophic and cannot be reactivated if the exogenous steroid is immediately withdrawn or if the dosage is insufficient to cope with a sudden stressful situation such as an infection. The longer the duration of the steroid therapy, the poorer is the ability of the adrenal gland to recover endogenous steroid secretion. Steroid therapy for a few weeks or months suppresses the adrenal cortex, but the gland can generally respond fairly promptly to endogenous (or exogenous) corticotropin.

After three months or so of steroid treatment (though actually probably not until after a year or more of therapy), the ability of the pituitary-adrenal axis to respond to stress is impaired. Following five or more years of supraphysiological doses of steroids, a permanent state of adrenal atrophy may be induced (especially in children, in whom this may occur after less than five years). This is iatrogenic Addison's disease. After long-term steroid therapy, the CRH-releasing mechanism in the hypothalamus is impaired, as well as the responsiveness of the adrenal cortex.

When steroid therapy is to be discontinued in patients who have received more than three months of treatment, it should be withdrawn slowly—the more slowly the longer the patient has been on the drug. A rate of withdrawal of prednisone of about 1 mg a week should be satisfactory in this situation. If the steroid needs to be withdrawn more rapidly, for example when there is a peptic ulcer, it should not be done at more than twice this rate (1 mg every three days). Such a program does not take into account the factor of a flare-up of the colitis as a consequence of treatment withdrawal; suitable programs in this situation will be discussed later in this chapter.

The ability of the adrenal cortex to respond to stress is diminished for a period of time after withdrawal of long-term steroid therapy. Surgical operations and intercurrent infections, and other medically stressful events such as myocardial infarction, need to be covered by additional steroid therapy, at a dosage of about 20 mg of prednisone or 100 mg of hydrocortisone daily.

Opinion varies about the length of time after steroid withdrawal for which supplemental steroids need to be given to patients subjected to operations and other stresses. Endocrinological studies have given periods varying from two weeks to two years for the duration of a diminished stress response following discontinuance of steroid therapy. The evidence favors the shorter period; so the authors suggest a compromise on two months after steroid withdrawal for all but the most major operations; one might be cautious and give a patient who has a major operation extra steroids up to a year after steroid withdrawal.

Although the long-term use of ACTH, rather than a steroid, allows the function of the adrenal gland to continue and the cortex does not atrophy, the hypothalamic CRH-releasing mechanism is still suppressed and it does not recover promptly. Thus it is illogical and of no help to change from an oral steroid to ACTH prior to discontinuing the steroid medication in order to obviate the effects of adrenal suppression.

PROGRAMS FOR THE USE OF SYSTEMIC STEROIDS

In general, patients with severe ulcerative colitis require a course of intravenous steroids; moderate colitis is an indication for oral steroids; and in mild colitis one can often rely on topical steroids or no steroids at all. A patient with a stubborn mild colitis may well benefit from a period on oral steroids, and one with a refractory moderate colitis may respond to intravenous medication. Except when there is relative rectal sparing, it is useful to add topical rectal steroids to a regimen involving oral or intravenous steroid treatment. The use of topical steroids is considered in a later section of this chapter.

The authors have stated a preference for prednisone (or prednisolone), over hydrocortisone and methylprednisolone, as the first-choice steroid; but they readily change from one to another as the need is indicated. Equivalent activity is provided by 5 mg of prednisone or prednisolone, 20 mg of hydrocortisone, and 4 mg of methylprednisolone.

Moderate Colitis

Although individual factors must be taken into account with each patient, the usual dosage of steroids in patients with ulcerative colitis of moderate severity, and in patients with mild cases being given oral steroids, is 20 mg of prednisone daily or its equivalent. Natural endogenous secretion of cortisol by the adrenal gland is greatest in the morning and lowest at night; so it is logical in these mild and moderate cases to obviate adrenal suppression by advising the patient to take the entire daily dose of prednisone in the morning. This probably helps to avoid sleeplessness, which may occur in patients who take therapeutic corticosteroids in the evening. More often than not, this dosage of steroids will be effective in causing the colitis to remit; and the response is judged clinically and by sigmoidoscopic examination. If recovery is prompt, with signs of inflammation disappearing from the rectal mucosa, a rule of thumb is to continue the prednisone at this dosage for six to eight weeks. If the response is slow, then the steroid needs to be continued for a longer period.

If there is no response or only a slight response, one should immediately try a larger dosage, such as 40 mg of prednisone daily divided into morning, noon, and evening doses, with a tendency to give more in the morning than later in the day. A daily dosage of 40 mg of prednisone should not be continued for more than two to three weeks after sigmoidoscopic examination shows remission. There is conflicting evidence on the efficacy of larger dosages of oral steroids. One report indicated no benefit from the use of 60 mg rather than 40 mg daily (64). The patient for whom 40 mg of oral prednisone daily is insufficient should be tried with a course of intravenous steroids. It is even the authors' feeling that patients who are not helped by 20 mg of prednisone daily should have a course of intravenous steroids.

Intravenous Steroids for Severe Colitis

In most medical centers with a wide experience of ulcerative colitis, patients with severe attacks are treated with a program of intravenous steroid medication. This is frequently combined with an intravenous antibiotic (chloramphenicol, tetracycline, or ampicillin is the choice of different experts, and this is discussed later in this chapter); and in many places the patient is kept on a totally intravenous regimen, avoiding oral feeding or restricting oral intake to an elemental diet. This is a regimen that "seems to work" in the hands of those treating patients with acute colitis in whom one is attempting to avoid colectomy (65), and it has been extrapolated for use in the moderate-to-severe case.

It is impossible to say whether all three aspects of the therapy—the steroid, the antibiotic, and bowel rest—are effective. There is satisfactory evidence for the effectiveness of the steroid. Those who rely on such a regimen are reluctant not to use all three aspects of it in an acute case; and they are unlikely to be able to prove or disprove statistically a benefit for bowel rest or for antibiotics in the treatment of patients who are not so severely ill. The possible reasons for the putative benefit of antibiotics are discussed later in this chapter. Withdrawal of oral feeding may be effective because a bacteriologically "cleaner" bowel results and enhances recovery; or because lack of stimulus for the gastrocolic reflex lowers the motor activity of the colon, encouraging healing; or because a dietary antigen, as yet unidentified, which may be causing a toxic immunological reaction in the colon in ulcerative colitis, is no longer being given (this is analogous to the recovery of the small intestinal mucosa in celiac disease following the withdrawal of gluten from the diet). All these are mostly speculations.

When the patient is dependent on intravenous hydration and alimentation, it is vital for the physician to ensure adequate prescription of sodium, potassium, water, calories, albumin, and blood. It is difficult to provide ideal alimentation through a peripheral venous catheter. Better alimentation requires a central venous catheter, but this has additional dangers—greater risks of infection and thrombosis, and risks of pulmonary damage during the insertion of the cannula. The various types of intravenous steroid regimen used in acute ulcerative colitis should only be employed for up to a week, and in this time no gross metabolic deficits should develop. For alimentation, 5% dextrose, 10% Intralipid, or a dilute amino acid mixture (such as Aminoplex-5, available in Britain) can be given into a peripheral vein and should be supportive until oral feeding can be started or until a decision is made to institute central venous alimentation. Patients with deficits of calcium and magnesium can be given these ions parenterally.

The forms of corticosteroid available for intravenous use are hydrocortisone, prednisolone sodium succinate, prednisolone-21-phosphate (these two prednisolone salts are supplied in doses with a prednisolone equivalent), and methylprednisolone. The authors normally give 40 to 60 mg of prednisolone daily, or 32 to 48 mg of methylprednisolone, in four divided doses, either as a slow infusion into the side-arm of a continuing intravenous drip or else mixed in one of the dextrose or saline infusion bottles. The dosage is according to the size of the patient and the severity of the disease, the larger dosage being prescribed for a 60 to 80-kg adult with severe colitis, the smaller dosage for a smaller person with less acute disease.

Such an intravenous steroid regimen can be used as a trial of medical therapy in patients with ulcerative colitis who may be destined for surgery. Lack of significant improvement within 48 hours or the development of toxic dilatation of the colon (or its lack of resolution) within 6 hours is an indication for immediate colectomy. The regimen should not be continued for more than five to seven days. If by this time there is improvement in the patient's condition and in the sigmoidoscopic appearance of the rectal mucosa, then oral feeding can be commenced. If there is no such improvement, then either this is an indication for surgery on account of the failure of medical therapy or else one might consider other measures that might be effective, such as changing the steroid, trying a different antibiotic, or resorting to a course of central venous alimentation with continuation of the intravenous steroid.

It is still debatable whether continuation of supportive parenteral alimentation and hyperalimentation is of any benefit in ulcerative colitis. There is little reason to think that its role is more than supportive while a natural recovery can take place. Such may be the case when there is an overwhelming emotional element in the flare-up of the colitis, which may be expected to abate as the patient has a few weeks of calm in a hospital environment.

On the whole, the patient whose severe ulcerative colitis has not shown improvement with five to seven days of intravenous steroid therapy and bowel rest will not be expected to do well, and it may be wisest to remove the colon at that time. On the other hand, total colectomy is such a drastic procedure that in treating the patient who is basically strong—the young patient rather than the older patient (although the surgery may be especially hazardous in the old and frail patient)—one can fairly safely persist, against the odds, with medical management, provided surgery is insisted upon if there is any deterioration.

If the intravenous regimen has been successful after five days or so of its use, the patient can be changed to oral steroids and oral feeding can be introduced. Clear liquids should be given for 24 to 48 hours, then a liquid diet for another one to three days, then a mechanically soft diet for a few more days, and then a full diet. The more the rectal mucosa is seen to have healed, the more rapid can be the progression to a full diet. The oral steroid dosage should be initially 40 mg of prednisone a day, or its equivalent. If the patient's response is satisfactory, this can be reduced by 5 mg daily every five days, down to a dosage of 20 mg of prednisone daily. If the recovery of the rectal mucosa has been complete, a faster rate of steroid reduction can be achieved, e.g., by 5 mg every three days. The patient should then be maintained on 20 mg of prednisone a day for a further six weeks before tailing off the steroids is considered.

Long-Term Use of Steroids

The long-term use of steroids is a matter about which some physicians hold strong feelings. It is associated with many of the undesirable side effects described in this chapter. These side effects are rarely troublesome in courses of steroids lasting three months or less. Repeated brief courses of steroids for recurrences of colitis are by no means as harmful with regard to side effects as is continuous steroid use. Adrenal gland suppression and tendencies to diabetes, hypertension, osteoporosis, and peptic ulceration are the most notable effects of long-term therapy. In children and prepubertal teenagers, chronic steroid administration of more than 7.5 mg of prednisone daily, or even of 7.5 mg daily, almost inevitably leads to stunting of growth and delay of pubertal development.

Truelove and his colleagues, in a controlled trial, showed that in the prevention of relapse there was no benefit in maintaining on steroid therapy patients with ulcerative colitis in remission (63). Only harm can come from this practice. The difficulty arises with the patient whose disease activity flares up whenever the steroid dosage is reduced. When this happens, it is usually when the dosage is down to 15 or 12.5 mg of prednisone daily.

The physician's skill is now tested, because if the patient has to be maintained on such a large dose of steroids, it will be better in many circumstances to advise a colectomy. One would tend to advise surgery more for patients who already have apparent steroid side effects, for prepubertal patients, for fit younger patients than for frail older patients, for patients whose recurrences of disease on lowering the steroid dosage were of moderate rather than of mild severity, and particularly for patients with more than a ten-year history of colitis extending proximal to the splenic flexure in whom there is a significant risk of developing cancer of the colon. One would tend away from advising surgery for patients in the early stages of the disease, and also for young adults who have not yet found a stable marriage and borne their family of children.

The important matter for the physician is to ascertain that the patient really is resistant to reduction of the steroid medication. Other aspects of the treatment program should be optimal. Is the patient receiving at least 2 gm daily of sulfasalazine? Has a larger dose of sulfasalazine, up to 4 gm, been tried? Are topical steroids being used effectively? Is the patient under emotional stresses that need to be dealt with? Are there any possible dietary manipulations? Usually there are no such manipulations that are known to be effective, but omission of fresh fruits and vegetables can be suggested. The patient may have hypolactasia and require a milk-free diet; a lactose tolerance test may be useful.

If attention has been paid to these factors, the patient can be tried with a second course of steroids, say 25 to 30 mg of prednisone daily, reducing to 20 mg after about two weeks, and then remaining at 20 mg for two months before a very slow further reduction is attempted. If this second course fails, or if the relapse following reduction of the steroid for the first time is of moderate severity, then the five-day intravenous steroid program can be used. Another thing to do is to change the steroid, e.g., from prednisone to hydrocortisone. Yet another course of action, which often is helpful, is to introduce azathioprine.

If none of these measures is successful, then the decision must be made as to whether to advise colectomy or to persist with chronic steroid administration. In the latter circumstance, the dosage can be reduced every six months or so to see if a remission can be maintained with less steroid. In ulcerative colitis, it is usually better in the long run for the patient to have a colectomy.

Alternate-Day Use of Steroids

In ulcerative colitis and in other diseases requiring the prescription of corticosteroids, the practice of giving a single dose on alternate days in order to lessen steroid side effects has been followed and continues to be followed by many physicians. There is no doubt that alternate-day steroid therapy is associated with fewer side effects and less adrenocortical suppression than a daily regimen of the same overall steroid dosage, although there may not be any less suppression of the hypothalamo-pituitary-adrenal axis. What appears to be the case, however, is that alternate-day steroid therapy is less effective in suppressing the disease than daily dosage. The lessening of side effects appears to parallel the lessening of the therapeutic effect, and so this is not a form of treatment that has good evidence in its favor. The published studies on ulcerative colitis do not show a controlled benefit from alternate-day use of steroids, and they show it to be particularly ineffectual in the acute stage. An exception to this pessimistic view seems to be in the case of prepubertal children, whose growth seems to proceed much better on an alternate-day steroid regimen than on a therapeutically equivalent daily steroid program.

TOPICAL STEROIDS

Steroids can be applied locally to the rectal mucosa, and this is an effective way of treating ulcerative colitis. Although some of the steroid is absorbed through the mucosa, a great deal of local benefit can be obtained for a small amount of systemic effect. It is estimated that approximately one-third of a locally applied dose will be systemically absorbed, and this can give rise to side effects and to adrenal suppression. Although this systemic absorption must be appreciated, the benefit:risk ratio is generally so good that topical steroids (up to 20 mg of prednisolone or 100 mg of hydrocortisone daily) can be regarded as a safe form of therapy in ulcerative colitis.

Hydrocortisone, prednisolone, and methylprednisolone are all available in various forms for topical use in the rectum. There are enemas (prepared and to be made up), suppositories, and foams.

Steroid Enemas

The steroid enemas are the most effective type of local steroid preparation. Cortenema is a 60-ml disposable, self-administered enema containing 100 mg of hydrocortisone in saline. In Britain, 20 mg of prednisolone is dissolved in 100 ml of normal saline in Predsol Retention Enemas; this dose is equivalent to that of Cortenema. The patient should attempt to retain the enema for at least 30 minutes (though there is benefit from briefer periods of retention) and preferably overnight. Medrol En-Pak (available in the United States from the Upjohn Company) is methylprednisolone acetate in 40-mg doses which are dissolved in up to 200 ml of warm water in a supplied administration set so that the enema can be given by slow infusion into the rectum. The amount of methylprednisolone in Medrol En-Pak is equivalent to approximately twice the dose of steroid contained in Cortenemas or Predsol enemas, and the greater volume allows the steroid to reach more proximal parts of the colon.

The rate of infusion should be roughly 100 ml per half hour. Such a slow rectal infusion can also be obtained by dissolving hydrocortisone hemisuccinate from ampules marketed for intravenous infusion in warm saline—100 mg of hydrocortisone in 100 ml of saline, or 200 mg of hydrocortisone in 200 ml of saline—in an intravenous infusion set with the plastic delivery end of the infusion set inserted gently through the anus. For these slow-infusion enemas, it is better if the foot of the patient's bed is elevated about 12 in so that the enema solution will pass proximally by gravity.

Steroid enemas should always be prescribed as part of the treatment of active ulcerative colitis, unless the condition is mild and restricted to the rectum, with normal mucosa visible beyond the sigmoidoscope. Patients with severe colitis should be given one Cortenema, or its equivalent, morning and night. For those with moderate colitis and with mild colitis extending proximal to the rectum, a once-daily dosage of the steroid enema should be prescribed, the patient being encouraged to take it at night before retiring. Just as physicians should insist that patients be compulsive about taking systemic steroid and antibiotic medications regularly without fail, so they should point out instances where it is not so vital to use a medication regularly. In mild ulcerative colitis, it should be in order for the patient to omit the steroid enema one night a week if taking it is inconvenient—for instance, if the patient is traveling.

Steroid enemas have been shown to be more effective than placebo enemas in ulcerative colitis, and the use of steroid enemas and oral steroids simultaneously is better than either alone (66). The steroid enemas will be less effective when disease affects the ascending colon. A 100-ml enema usually reaches to the splenic flexure.

When the dose of oral steroids is being reduced, the steroid enema should preferably be continued beyond the time when the oral steroid is finally discontinued; although if the patient protests inconvenience, the enema can be given on alternate days, or can be discontinued earlier if there is a complete and persistent remission of the colitis as seen on sigmoidoscopy. About two weeks after the oral steroids have been discontinued, the steroid enema can be limited to alternate nights for about a week, then to every third night for a while, and then it too can be discontinued.

Patients with mild colitis can be treated with steroid enemas and without oral steroids. Such patients should follow a strict daily (nightly) routine of one Cortenema or its equivalent for six to eight weeks before reducing the frequency of the enema administration in accordance with the sigmoidoscopic findings. If the rectal mucosa is at all inflamed, even mildly, a daily steroid enema (with occasional omissions) should be continued. There are some patients who need continual treatment with steroid enemas. The absorption of 30 mg of hydrocortisone a day is no great hazard, and the enemas can be used indefinitely if necessary. Every six months or so, a reduction in enema frequency should be attempted. Since the enemas in these circumstances are being used more to reduce the patient's symptoms than to help his overall health (although the enemas should help prevent iron deficiency anemia), the enemas can be omitted on two successive days each week in the hope that this may minimize adrenocortical suppression (though this may not be so).

Patients receiving daily steroid enemas should be considered to need steroid supplements to cover surgical operations or other traumas during their treatment with the enemas or within two months afterwards.

Steroid Suppositories

For patients with mild ulcerative colitis confined to the distal 10 cm of the rectum (usually designated as ulcerative proctitis), a suppository of prednisolone or hydrocortisone inserted into the rectum for slow dissolution can be an effective local form of steroid therapy. Twenty-five-milligram hydrocortisone suppositories and 5-mg suppositories of prednisolone-21-phosphate are available and are of equivalent therapeutic activity. These suppositories can be the sole form of therapy in such mild colitis, although oral sulfasalazine can be added to the regimen if the response to the suppositories is not prompt.

Steroid suppositories containing less than these amounts of steroid, which often contain added local anesthetics, lubricants, and anti-infectious agents, are not intended for the treatment of ulcerative colitis.

Steroid Foam

Hydrocortisone acetate is available in a 10% foam, marketed as Cortifoam. One application supplies approximately 90 mg of hydrocortisone in the rectum. Cortifoam can be used as the local steroid preparation by patients with mild ulcerative colitis extending up to about 15 to 20 cm from the anus.

SULFASALAZINE

Sulfasalazine, also known as salicylazosulfapyridine and sold as Azulfidine and SAS-500 in the United States and as Salazopyrin in Britain, is a compound of 5-aminosalicylic acid with sulfapyridine. Together with the corticosteroids, it is one of the two definitely effective forms of drug therapy in ulcerative colitis, although the circumstances of its benefit differ from those of the corticosteroids. Sulfasalazine appears to be effective in mild and moderate rather than in severe colitis and is useful in quiescent colitis in preventing relapses of the disease.

In the early days of the sulfonamides (around 1940), 5-aminosalicylic acid was compounded with sulfapyridine in the hope that this might be a helpful form of treatment for rheumatoid arthritis. Patients with rheumatoid disease were not helped; but is was noticed that in patients with arthritis in association with ulcerative colitis, the bowel disease improved. Sulfasalazine has thus been in use in treating ulcerative colitis since the early 1940s—ten years longer than cortisone.

Therapeutic Benefit

The trials of sulfasalazine that have shown its benefit in ulcerative colitis have mostly been with outpatients, mainly those with mild, moderate, or quiescent disease, rather than severe disease. Sulfasalazine may not be particularly effective in treating severe colitis, and this fact may have a scientific basis in the pharmacokinetics of sulfasalazine. The drug is broken down into its salicylate and sulfonamide components only by the flora of the colon. It is barely absorbed and is inactive until it reaches the colon. This explains its specific action in ulcerative colitis. There have been recent observations that there is less colonic breakdown of the drug in diarrheal states, which include those found in severe ulcerative colitis (67).

Several well-controlled trials have shown that sulfasalazine taken continually by patients with ulcerative colitis in remission is extremely effective in preventing relapses of the disease. In the study by Dissanayake and Truelove (68), 13% of patients taking 500 mg of sulfasalazine four times daily relapsed in a six-month period, compared with a 56% relapse rate in patients taking a placebo tablet of similar appearance. This study showed that sulfasalazine was as effective in preventing relapse three years or more after the last attack of colitis as it was when the last attack was more recent.

Side Effects

Sulfasalazine does have side effects that limit its use. In patients who do not experience these side effects, the drug can and should be continued indefinitely. Fortunately, most of the side effects of sulfasalazine are apparent when they occur (unlike the progression to diabetes, hypertension, and osteoporosis with continued steroid administration), at least as far as we know. They can be listed as follows:

1. *Nausea* and sometimes *vomiting:* Some patients find sulfasalazine too nauseating to take. They should be encouraged to persist because these symptoms often settle down after about two weeks' use. Patients with organic dyspepsia, for instance with peptic ulcer disease or esophageal reflux, should not persist with the treatment if they get symptoms, as they often do. However, there is no evidence that sulfasalazine actually exacerbates either peptic ulcers or reflux esophagitis.

2. *Skin rashes:* The sulfonamide component of sulfasalazine is responsible for a wide variety of skin rashes due to hypersensitivity. These can be macular, papular or pustular, irritating or nonirritating. Photosensitive rashes can occur, as can erythema nodosum. In patients with active ulcerative colitis, the rashes need to be distinguished from rashes of the colitis, such as the pustular eruption of pyoderma gangrenosum and such as erythema nodosum, which is more likely to be due to the colitis itself. A dangerous exfoliative dermatitis, which has been known to be fatal, has been described (fortunately, rarely) following the use of sulfasalazine. Except in this latter condition, which is an indication for systemic steroids, all that is required in sulfasalazine hypersensitivity is to withdraw the drug.

3. *Blood dyscrasias:* Blood dyscrasias are the most troublesome side effects of sulfasalazine because they usually develop more insidiously than nausea and skin rashes; and they can, very rarely, be fatal. The commonest is hemolytic anemia. This can be mild, in the form of contracted red cells and Heinz body formation without an actual anemia, but it can be more severe (43). Mild forms of this hemolytic anemia are very common with large doses of the drug and generally remit upon reduction of the dosage. Patients with glucose-6-phosphate dehydrogenase (G-6-PD) deficiency exhibit a hemolytic state when they are given a number of drugs, including sulfasalazine. The granulocytes and

the platelets can also be affected by sulfasalazine therapy. Agranulocytosis, thrombocytopenia, and a pancytopenia of red cells, granulocytes, and platelets together have all been reported. Sulfasalazine inhibits folic acid absorption from the small intestine and can cause a megaloblastic anemia due to folic acid deficiency (44). Patients receiving sulfasalazine should be checked for folic acid deficiency and may need to be maintained on 1 mg of supplementary folic acid daily.

4. *Arthralgias:* Joint aches and muscle aches occur from time to time in patients receiving sulfasalazine. These must be distinguished from arthritis due to ulcerative colitis, which is commoner and more marked; but the distinction is sometimes not possible to make except by discontinuing the sulfasalazine.

5. *Headache:* Some patients receiving sulfasalazine experience headaches, which usually remit after a few days' use of the drug.

6. *Orange-colored urine:* This causes no discomfort or danger to the patient, but sometimes patients are alarmed when they notice it. The color is due to the sulfapyridine.

7. *Pulmonary infiltration:* This has been reported, rarely, in patients taking long term sulfasalazine.

Should rashes, granulocytopenia, thrombocytopenia, hypoplastic anemia, severe hemolytic anemia, any degree of G-6-PD deficiency anemia, or arthritis develop in patients on sulfasalazine therapy, these patients should always in future avoid the drug. Patients with severe rashes or with blood dyscrasias should also avoid all other sulfonamides.

Dosage

The incidence of side effects in patients taking sulfasalazine increases markedly with increasing dosage. In the controlled trials of the prevention of relapse, the dosage used has generally been 2 gm daily. Side effects are uncommon at this dosage, whereas they are common with dosages of 4 gm daily, and especially with more than 4 gm daily. The 2-gm dosage is the smallest that any trial has shown to be effective, although a 1.5-gm dosage is probably effective if the patient cannot tolerate 2 gm.

There are conflicting views on the use of larger dosages, although it is agreed that 4 gm daily should not be exceeded. Das and Eastwood and their coworkers correlated relapse in their patients with low serum levels of sulfapyridine and concluded that a larger dosage is more effective than a smaller dosage, in the range of 2 to 4 gm daily (69). On the other hand, Azad Khan and Truelove (67) found that patients who had an adequate serum level of sulfapyridine while the disease was in remission and they were taking 2 gm of sulfasalazine daily had a lower level when they relapsed. The conclusion of Azad Khan and Truelove was the opposite of that of Das and Eastwood; that is, it seemed that patients with active disease had lower sulfapyridine levels as a result of their disease activity, rather than the other way around. Patients with diarrhea appear to have a diminished bacterial breakdown of sulfasalazine in the colon.

The authors' recommendation in this book is based on these observations, and it is that the 2-gm daily dosage should be used initially in mild and moderate cases and the 4-gm dose in severe cases. (If patients with severe colitis are not breaking down the sulfasalazine, they should not be as liable to side effects.)

When patients taking 2 gm of sulfasalazine daily prove to be resistant to reduction of steroid dosage, then a 4-gm regimen can be tried. Any patient taking 4 gm who has mild side effects such as nausea or a mild hemolytic anemia (not due to G-6-PD deficiency) can be lowered to a 2-gm regimen. Of course, 3 gm daily can be prescribed for situations in between those for which 2 or 4 gm is being recommended.

Blood levels of the sulfasalazine breakdown products demonstrate a 6 to 8-hour duration in the blood. This indicates that the drug should probably be given in four six-hourly doses of 0.5 or 1 gm.

The Mechanism of Action of Sulfasalazine

It remains somewhat of a mystery how sulfasalazine works in patients with ulcerative colitis, beyond the knowledge that colonic microbial breakdown of the drug to 5-aminosalicylic acid and sulfapyridine is required. It seems likely that the beneficial effect is a local one due either to the salicylate or to the sulfonamide. Salicylates and sulfonamides on their own have not been shown to afford any significant benefit in ulcerative colitis, and a compound of 5-aminosalicylic acid and sulfadimidine was ineffective in one study (70). One can only speculate as to whether it is the salicylate or the sulfonamide that is the effective moiety, although some synergistic effect of the two cannot be ruled out. Since the only other effective medications in ulcerative colitis are the corticosteroids and azathioprine (the latter only marginally effective), and these are both immunosuppressive agents, and since salicylates, but not sulfonamides or other antibiotics, are beneficial in autoimmune diseases such as rheumatoid arthritis and rheumatic fever, the guess of the authors is that sulfasalazine is more likely to act through its salicylate than through its sulfonamide component in ulcerative colitis. There is recent evidence that sulfasalazine may be effective in ulcerative colitis by virtue of an inhibition of prostaglandin synthesis, which is a known action of salicylates (71). There have also been recent reports that sulfasalazine and 5-aminosalicylate enemas are effective in ulcerative colitis but sulfapyridine enemas are ineffective.

AZATHIOPRINE (IMURAN)

Azathioprine is a drug that suppresses immune responses in a manner that is not well understood. It is used to inhibit the immune processes of rejection following homologous transplantation of organs. It has been tried in treating a number of autoimmune diseases, including Crohn's disease and ulcerative colitis. The experience of its use in ulcerative colitis allows one to say that it has some effect, although a small one, in treating ulcerative colitis.

The results of two recently published reports of trials indicate that azathioprine has a positive effect on ulcerative colitis: 1) in allowing a smaller dose of steroids to be used than would otherwise be the case for a given therapeutic effect of the steroid (72); 2) as maintenance therapy in maintaining remission for a year after an attack of ulcerative colitis (though not after the first attack of the disease), the benefit here being on the border line of the 5% significance level (73); and 3) in improving, marginally, the sigmoidoscopic appearances and the degree of activity as indicated by rectal biopsy specimens after one month of treatment for an attack of the disease (73).

Dosage

The current dosage recommendation for azathioprine is 2 mg per kg of body weight, or 100 to 200 mg daily. The 50-mg tablets can be taken two to four times daily. In the trials reported in treating ulcerative colitis, this dosage has not been associated with significant side effects.

Side Effects

As an immunosuppressant, azathioprine does have potentially dangerous side effects. There is marrow depression, which is fairly common but nearly always reversible on withdrawal of the drug; the marrow depression can give rise to an increased incidence of infections. Patients receiving azathioprine should have a weekly blood count (including counts for red cells, white cells, and platelets) for the first month of treatment, and this can be done subsequently every two or three weeks. The patient should be warned that if an infection, a sore throat, or a fever should develop, the drug should not be taken and the physician should be informed. The drug should be discontinued and not used again if there is any sign of marrow suppression, although it is sometimes safe when the cytopenia is only very mild to reduce the dose of the azathioprine and to observe the blood count over the next few days, continuing the drug if the blood count recovers.

Azathioprine is metabolized by the liver, and a smaller dose should be used in patients with a diseased liver. The drug is hepatotoxic itself, occasionally causing a hepatocellular or a cholestatic jaundice. Transaminase levels in the blood should be checked in the first few weeks of treatment and every few months thereafter; a rise in transaminase levels that is ascribed to the drug rather than to underlying liver disease is an indication for withdrawal of azathioprine.

A third important side effect of azathioprine is pancreatitis, which, interestingly, is also a reported side effect of steroids and of sulfasalazine. In a recent trial of azathioprine in treating Crohn's disease, there were two instances of acute pancreatitis in a fairly small series (74).

Other undesirable side effects include alopecia and rashes. Long-term administration of azathioprine in other diseases (admittedly at larger doses than 2 mg per kg of body weight) has given rise to a disproportionate incidence in the development of malignant tumors, particularly reticulum cell sarcomas. Also, damage to the germinal cells is a theoretical risk of long-term treatment.

Despite these side effects, using azathioprine may be no less safe than using steroids in dosages of 20 mg daily of prednisone, or more, over periods exceeding six months. Azathioprine is probably fairly safe when used in the dosages suggested and with the patients having frequent blood tests, at least in courses of up to two years (when the oncogenic potential may still be insignificant).

Indications and Contraindications

The authors confine the use of azathioprine to patients who have been receiving systemic steroids for more than three months in whom the colitis cannot be controlled by less than 15 mg of prednisone daily, and to other patients who are experiencing troublesome side effects of steroids. An effective larger dose of steroids is then reinstituted, with the addition of azathioprine; and after two to four weeks of improvement on this regimen, the dosage of the steroid is progressively reduced, aiming at 10 mg of prednisone daily, if not a complete withdrawal of the steroid. After one year of azathioprine, the dosage that is being used is halved for a month or two before withdrawing the azathioprine, in the hope that a remission is maintained. If the patient then relapses, one is prepared to reintroduce the azathioprine, balancing the risks of the drug against those of alternative courses of action.

The authors are hesitant, but not especially reluctant if there is good indication, to use azathioprine in children and in adults who have not yet completed their families. The harmful effects of azathioprine on the germinal tissue are more theoretical than observed, and azathioprine does not have the growth-stunting effect that steroids certainly have. Large doses of steroids may be just as harmful to the genes as azathioprine. Nevertheless, the authors would not use azathioprine in young patients unless the only alternatives were large doses of steroids or total colectomy, a fact that probably also applies to patients in other age groups. Also, the authors would regard the drug as being contraindicated in the pregnant and potentially pregnant woman; and they would be prepared to accede to a request for abortion if a patient taking azathioprine became pregnant and did not want the child or was in any way apprehensive about the possible teratogenicity of the drug.

OTHER IMMUNOSUPPRESSIVE AGENTS

Another immunosuppressant drug, 6-mercaptopurine, has been used in treating ulcerative colitis (in dosages of 50 to 150 mg daily) with encouraging results (75). There have been no controlled trials, and experience with 6-mercaptopurine is not as wide as with azathioprine. The drug 6-mercaptopurine causes marrow suppression and at present seems to offer no advantages over azathioprine.

Other approaches to immunosuppressive therapy may be developed. There has been a report of the use of horse antilymphocyte serum in two patients with ulcerative colitis, one of whom appeared to respond to the treatment (76).

ANTIBIOTICS AND OTHER ANTIBACTERIAL DRUGS

The usefulness of antibiotics in treating ulcerative colitis has never been well evaluated. There is no evidence to date that ulcerative colitis is caused by a bacterial agent, and so the use of antibacterial drugs is theoretically illogical. On the other hand, it may be of help in the treatment of ulcerative colitis to inhibit the colonic bacterial flora in some way. Antibiotics are certainly indicated when a septicemia complicates severe ulcerative colitis and when there is perforation, peritonitis, or abscess formation (though in the latter circumstances surgery is the treatment of choice); hence, it may be logical to prescribe a broad-spectrum antibiotic for patients with severe colitis as prophylaxis against potential septicemia.

Sulfasalazine is effective in ulcerative colitis, and it is possible that this is due to its sulfonamide component and therefore to its antibacterial activity. Only one out of several studies has shown any consistent suppression of the fecal flora in patients with ulcerative colitis treated with sulfasalazine (77).

In practice, however, many leading centers treating ulcerative colitis use a broad-spectrum antibiotic in severe cases. Ampicillin, tetracycline (65), chloramphenicol, and, in previous years, penicillin with streptomycin have all been recommended for parenteral use in patients with severe acute ulcerative colitis.

If the rationale is to suppress the colonic flora, then one should aim to inhibit the anaerobic *Bacteroides fragilis* and the coliform bacteria. Most effective for this would be a combination of clindamycin and gentamicin, but clindamycin is particularly likely to induce another form of colitis, membranous colitis (which can also occur as a result of using other broad-spectrum antibiotics, including tetracycline). In one study, the combination of clindamycin with gentamicin was associated with a greater incidence of membranous colitis than when clindamycin was used alone (78). One can speculate that to inhibit the colonic flora too efficiently might lead to some harmful change in the proportions of the remaining species. One is left, therefore, with the empirical practices of the various experts. Oral antibiotics can actually exacerbate ulcerative colitis, and ampicillin has been observed to do this. However, ampicillin is used widely as a prophylactic antibiotic in acute ulcerative colitis.

This leaves chloramphenicol, which in extended oral courses is known to cause a fatal aplastic anemia in about 1 person in 20,000 (as well as a more frequent reversible marrow suppression); and tetracycline, which is active against only about 50% of strains of *Bacteroides fragilis,* often causes a phlebitis, and, rarely, is toxic to the liver and kidneys. The risks of these drugs are probably much less than the potential risks of an acute attack of severe ulcerative colitis; so it is the authors' practice to administer one or the other. The dosages used are: for chloramphenicol, 50 mg per kg of body weight daily in four divided doses intravenously for five days only; and for tetracycline, 1 gm daily in four divided slow intravenous boluses.

When there is evidence of bacteremic shock, the choice of antibiotics must be such as to inhibit all the organisms that may be contributing to this state. The results of blood cultures are usually not available for 24 hours or more. Severe hypotension, inappropriate to the degree of blood and fluid loss, is the principal sign of gram-negative shock. The three antibiotics gentamicin, clindamycin, and a cephalosporin such as cefazolin should be used together in this situation. The risks of membranous colitis are small in relation to the dangers of septicemic shock.

In the management of moderate colitis and resistant forms of mild colitis, antibiotics are sometimes prescribed, especially when sulfasalazine cannot be used because of the occurrence of side effects.

The benefit of sulfasalazine is so marked that one feels that one must strive to reproduce its effect with another preparation if sulfasalazine itself cannot be used. Other sulfonamides are the most logical and the most popular, and those used are phthalylsulfathiazole (Sulfathalidine), 1 gm three times daily, and sulfisoxazole, 1 gm three or four times daily. On many occasions, the hypersensitivity to sulfasalazine applies to all sulfonamides, and so long-term ampicillin has been used. The authors would be reluctant to recommend ampicillin, but it may be worth trying the sulfonamides, because they have not been known to exacerbate the colitis. There are insufficient studies yet to prove them worthless, and one might benefit the patient without the risk of doing much harm.

There has been one favorable report of the use of a trimethoprim-sulfonamide combination in treating ulcerative colitis (79). Trimethoprim, 80 mg, and sulfamethoxazole, 400 mg, are combined in a single tablet, now generically known as cotrimoxazole and marketed as Bactrim or Septra (Septrin in Britain); the usual dosage is two tablets every 12 hours; double-strength tablets are now available. This form of treatment has had no formal study in ulcerative colitis, and so its effectiveness cannot be assessed.

Metronidazole (Flagyl), an antiprotozoal drug which is also active against *Bacteroides fragilis,* is being used at one or two medical centers in the treatment of Crohn's disease. There is no evidence of its value in ulcerative colitis, and its long-term use has been complicated by a peripheral neuropathy.

CROMOLYN (DISODIUM CROMOGLYCATE)

Disodium cromoglycate (cromolyn) has been used for a number of years in the treatment of asthma and hay fever. Particles of the compound are inhaled onto the mucous membrane, where they stabilize the mast cells, preventing the release of histamine in response to antigenic stimulation. Ulcerative colitis is primarily a mucosal disease, and it seems that cromolyn applied to the colonic mucosa benefits patients with ulcerative colitis. A positive effect has been observed in two controlled studies, one in which cromolyn was given by enema for ulcerative colitis limited to the rectum (80), and the other in which cromolyn was given by mouth for mild but more extensive ulcerative colitis (81). The oral route is effective because there is no breakdown of the drug in the gastrointestinal tract. The oral dosage used was 2 gm daily, but 200 mg four times daily is now the recommended dosage. There is no information yet to say whether it should be given continuously or for courses of just a few weeks.

One can see the place cromolyn would have in the management of ulcerative colitis. It would be most valuable in patients with mild or moderate (but not severe) colitis, resistant to topical steroids or to moderate doses of oral steroids. Cromolyn will probably not replace or even supplement the steroids for severe cases; and for limited distal colitis, the efficacy and lack of risk of topical steroids may not affect the role of these as the first line of therapy. Cromolyn may prove to be an alternative to sulfasalazine as maintenance therapy to prevent relapses of ulcerative colitis in remission. It has recently been marketed in Britain as Nalcrom. The only side effect reported has been nausea in some patients. However, one of the authors has observed exacerbation of conjunctivitis when cromolyn was successfully causing the colitis to remit.

Cromolyn is a rather expensive drug.

RESUSCITATIVE MEASURES

Severe Colitis

The general principles of resuscitative and supportive therapy apply to patients with severe ulcerative colitis. These patients may lose sodium, chloride, potassium, and water, and blood and protein, all of which must be replaced appropriately. Frequent observations of plasma electrolytes and plasma protein levels and of the hemoglobin and hematocrit concentrations are essential in monitoring these parameters. The patient may become shocked as a result of blood and fluid loss; and so the blood pressure and the central venous pressure may be appropriate indexes to observe. Blood loss is sometimes aggravated by a lack of clotting factors. This can be detected by measurement of the prothrombin time, the partial thromboplastin time, and other clotting tests. Factor VIII and some other clotting factors are now available for replacement therapy.

Shock may also be the result of septicemia, and this requires fluid replacement, with central venous pressure monitoring, large doses of steroids, and the broadest possible antibiotic cover. The shocked patient is nearly always hypoxic and acidotic, and the blood gases and pH must be followed and treated appropriately with oxygen and bicarbonate. Hypoxia can also develop in patients with ulcerative colitis as a result of pulmonary emboli, to which colitic patients have a disposition; as a result of myopericarditis (which is a rare peripheral manifestation of ulcerative colitis) (49); as a result of a rare pulmonary infiltration which has been reported in association with ulcerative colitis (46); as a result of pulmonary infiltration due to sulfasalazine therapy; as a result of atelectasis developing in patients confined to bed; and as a result of preexistent pulmonary or cardiac disease (which is in fact more likely than the specific associations with ulcerative colitis).

The patient with severe ulcerative colitis has the best chance of recovery from the attack and of responding to the specific measures such as steroids if his physiological parameters are as normal as possible. It is wise to add a parenteral multiple vitamin supplement if there has been any suggestion of malnutrition.

Moderate and Mild Colitis

It is also important in ulcerative colitis of lesser severity to ensure that the patient's physiological modalities are optimal. The colitis does not have to be severe for electrolyte abnormalities and dehydration to occur, and these must be corrected. Malnutrition and hypoproteinemia are generally indicative of moderate rather than mild colitis, but anemia can develop even in the mildest forms. Steroids themselves are catabolic, and their mineralocorticoid effect causes potassium depletion. The patient's recovery and the response to the specific drugs will be enhanced if hypoproteinemia and anemia are corrected.

The patient must be encouraged to eat a plentiful and nutritious diet and to achieve a good weight for his or her height. Young women who prefer to remain slim (not an unusual preference in patients who have lost weight as a result of gastrointestinal disease) must be convinced that while their colitis is active their health will be improved by their being better nourished. It is the authors' impression that the undernourished patient does not show cushingoid effects from steroid treatment and that this indicates that the patient is not receiving the maximum benefit from that form of treatment.

Correction of Anemia

The causes of the anemia that is common in patients with ulcerative colitis have been listed in Chapter 8. The most usual form is an iron deficiency anemia. Oral iron preparations have a tendency to inflame the colon in ulcerative colitis. Therefore, hematological results that indicate an iron deficiency state without there being an actual anemia should be noted, but the anemia should not be corrected. A hemoglobin level below 11.0 to 11.5 gm per 100 ml or a hematocrit below 33 to 35% is an indication for iron supplements. Oral ferrous gluconate or ferrous fumarate should be tried first; but if the patient has any adverse effects from the iron, or if there is a history of intolerance to oral iron, or if the colitis remains unduly active during oral iron treatment, then oral preparations should not be used. Weekly or twice-weekly injections of intramuscular iron should be used whenever the hemoglobin drops below 10.5 gm per 100 ml or so, or the hematocrit below about 31%. Intravenous parenteral iron is another alternative. Iron deficiency anemia resistant to oral and parenteral iron administration frequently requires blood transfusions for its correction, although one must be sure that there is no other basis to the anemia.

Vitamin B_{12} and folic acid deficiency are common in patients with Crohn's disease; but in ulcerative colitis, folic acid deficiency often develops as a result of dietary restriction or from sulfasalazine therapy. Folic acid and vitamin B_{12} deficiency are not uncommon in the community and so ought to be checked if a patient with ulcerative colitis develops an anemia.

The hemolytic anemia that has been described as an association with ulcerative colitis requires specific treatment of the colitis and should respond to steroids. Hemolytic anemia caused by sulfasalazine therapy is treated by stopping that drug or, if the anemia is mild and there is no G-6-PD deficiency, by reducing the dosage. Anemia resulting from azathioprine-induced bone marrow depression is an indication for discontinuing the azathioprine. The anemia of chronic disease that can occur in active ulcerative colitis can only be dealt with by treatment of the primary disease or by blood transfusion. In patients with any severe anemia in ulcerative colitis (hemoglobin less than 9 gm per 100 ml or hematocrit less than 28%), blood should be transfused to achieve a normal hemoglobin level, unless there is a rapid response of the anemia to steroids or to drug withdrawal. The more ill the patient, the more necessary is the blood transfusion.

Restoration of Nutrition

Elemental Diets

A patient with severe colitis is often nauseous and intolerant of large meals. If there has been weight loss, it is important to restore the weight by high-calorie and high-protein feeding. This can be achieved by supplementing solid food with some of the elemental diets that contain amino acids, monosaccharide sugars, and short-chain fatty acids. Those now on the market include Vivonex, Ensure, and Precision Isotonic. They all contain various electrolyte and vitamin supplements. The manufacturers' literature should be consulted for their composition and caloric value and for their osmolarity. Many are hypertonic, and this may not be well tolerated by the patient. Some contain lactose and should probably be avoided in ulcerative colitis for that reason, particularly if there is a question of hypolactasia.

The diet can also be supplemented by parenteral feeding. The peripheral veins can be used for giving lipid preparations (Intralipid) and dilute sugar and amino acid infusions. It is difficult to provide more than 1,000 calories per day by these means.

Parenteral Hyperalimentation

On the other hand, the use of a central venous catheter through which greater amounts of calories and amino acids can be infused is associated with significant risks of infection, thrombosis, and lung injury. In view of these risks, such a restorative nutritional measure in ulcerative colitis can only be justified in patients who are 20% or more below their ideal body weight and who require colectomy, which would be hazardous in such a malnourished person. If the surgery can safely be held over for a few weeks, parenteral hyperalimentation can be used as a supplementary or sole means of nutritional resuscitation; however, there are only a very limited number of patients with ulcerative colitis in whom it should be used. In most patients requiring colectomy to control their disease, the catabolic effects of the continued presence of the colon more than outweigh the anabolic benefits of parenteral hyperalimentation.

There are two instances in which parenteral hyperalimentation can be used in ulcerative colitis. First, there is the grossly malnourished patient with chronically active disease whose mucosal inflammation is less than in the severe category, who has reached the point at which colectomy is required but in whom the operation is not urgent. Second, there is the patient who has not responded fully, or even at all, to five to seven days of intravenous steroids with peripheral alimentation but in whom one would wish, after careful thought, to attempt to avoid surgery. Four to six weeks of hyperalimentation can then be instituted, watching at all times for indications to discontinue the medical program and to proceed to immediate surgery. The wisdom of this approach is influenced by the likelihood of a remission in such a patient; if remission is perceived to be unlikely, then the risks of the parenteral hyperalimentation are not worth taking.

Sometimes the patient is so adamantly opposed to colectomy that the physician can offer the hope of avoidance of the operation with a trial of parenteral hyperalimentation, provided that physician and patient are aware of and are prepared to accept probable additional risks. The physician should rarely allow himself to be influenced by his patient contrary to his better judgment; but in cases of resistant moderate-to-severe ulcerative colitis, one can often, fairly safely, buy time to persuade the patient that his disease can only be dealt with successfully by colectomy and that afterwards he will feel so much better. Many patients nowadays insist on trying every form of medical treatment reported in newspapers before agreeing to total colectomy. The occasional successes with parenteral hyperalimentation in ulcerative colitis are often in patients in whom there has been a great emotional component in their clinical picture, and the hyperalimentation regimen is supportive while they are in hospital and while a slow, natural remission of the disease occurs. Generally, though, the effectiveness of parenteral hyperalimentation in managing ulcerative colitis has been disappointing.

Parenteral hyperalimentation should only be used in medical centers already experienced in this procedure. One can begin one's experience with this form of therapy with patients with more clear-cut indications than those with ulcerative colitis. The technique will not be described here: appropriate reviews should be consulted (82). Hypertonic carbohydrate and amino acid solutions, alternated with lipid solutions, are infused via a subclavian venous catheter. A positive nitrogen balance should be attained. All known electrolytes, minerals, and vitamins that are required should be supplied in correct amounts.

The risks are as follows: pneumothorax and pulmonary contusion during introduction of the catheter, this sometimes being followed by pulmonary infection; infection of the catheter from the skin site leading to systemic and metastatic infection, this being minimized by meticulous aseptic techniques in the insertion and care of the cannula; thrombosis in the subclavian vein; acute hyperglycemia resulting from the quantity of glucose infused; and acute fatty liver from excessively rapid glucose feeding—this can develop within a week and is less common with the use of lipid solutions in the alimentation regimen. Indications of fatty liver are a rise in the serum transaminases and the reporting of pain by the patient over the area of the liver, which may become enlarged. The treatment of fatty liver is to reduce the amount of carbohydrate being given. Other metabolic complications, e.g., hypocalcemia and hypomagnesemia, should be avoidable; but they commonly occur, as a manifestation of our incomplete knowledge of the true requirements for parenteral alimentation. Other rare problems that can occur are breaking off of part of the catheter, perforation of the pericardium, and air embolism; any of these can cause severe morbidity. When infective or thrombotic complications occur, the parenteral hyperalimentation must be discontinued, even if this means that the operation that was to have been avoided must now take place.

SYMPTOMATIC MEASURES

Normalization of Bowel Habit

The diseased colon is liable to have disordered motor function, so that patients with ulcerative colitis, both active and in remission, have many features of the irritable colon syndrome. As a result, they may suffer from constipation or diarrhea, or both alternately. Diarrhea that appears explicable on the basis of active inflammation may also have a component of increased motor activity. Patients with a distal proctitis may become constipated as a result of inhibiting their stool movements for fear of aggravating their rectal symptoms. In brief, the patient with ulcerative colitis can be helped by relief of diarrhea and constipation, aside from the use of anti-inflammatory medications.

For diarrhea without cramping abdominal pains and without episodes of constipation, diphenoxylate (Lomotil), 2.5 mg, one or two tablets four times daily, should be tried. A stronger antidiarrheal medication is codeine, 15 mg, four times daily. An alternative to diphenoxylate that seems to have a similar mode of action and may have some advantages in producing fewer side effects is the new drug loperamide (Imodium), 2 mg being roughly equivalent to 2.5 mg of diphenoxylate. If there is also abdominal pain and constipation and the picture resembles the irritable colon syndrome, the use of a mild tranquilizer and an antispasmodic is appropriate. As a tranquilizer, phenobarbital, 15 mg, two to four times daily, is suitable; or diazepam (Valium), 5 mg. As an antispasmodic, belladonna, 8 mg taken just before meals and at bedtime, is the first choice; propantheline bromide (Pro-Banthine), 15 mg, is stronger and more likely to cause the side effects of dryness, blurred vision, and urinary retention. There are useful combination tablets of phenobarbital with belladonna and phenobarbital with propantheline.

Constipated patients, and many patients with diarrhea, benefit from the use of a hydrophilic preparation to form a soft bulky stool which can regularize their bowel habit. Psyllium and methylcellulose preparations are suitable. Psyllium is available in Metamucil and in Effersyllium (Normacol Special in Britain). Dioctyl sodium sulfosuccinate is supplied as Colace and as Surfak (Dioctyl-Medo in Britain), and combined with methylcellulose in Dialose. Methylcellulose is supplied alone in Britain in Iso-Gel. A suggested dosage is 5 ml of Metamucil nightly or twice daily. Paraffin preparations are not advised, and pharmacological laxatives such as senna, cascara, and bisacodyl should be avoided in patients with ulcerative colitis.

There are two cautions to be stated with regard to the use of these symptomatic agents in ulcerative colitis. First, they should not be used as an alternative to specific therapy of the colitis and not without proper evaluation of the disease, including a sigmoidoscopy. Second, the opiates and the codeine drugs and the anticholinergics should not be used in acute colitis, when they have been known to precipitate toxic dilatation of the colon.

Relief of Pain

The foremost rule for the relief of pain in patients with ulcerative colitis is to ascertain its cause and to treat that cause. Abdominal pain that is arising from an inflamed bowel should respond to suppression of the inflammation. Pain that is due to a pericolic abcess or to peritonitis needs to be treated urgently by surgery. If the abdominal pain is greater than the degree of colitis would indicate, then it is assumed to be due to abnormal colonic motility and requires treatment with antispasmodics and is usually also helped by a mild tranquilizer and a stool softener (the combination of phenobarbital, belladonna, and psyllium is a useful regimen).

One must be sure that the pain is not due to another organic cause of abdominal pain, bearing in mind that renal calculi are especially frequent in patients with ulcerative colitis. Pain can be a sign of the development of carcinoma of the colon complicating ulcerative colitis. Abdominal pain must always be fully investigated before resorting to treatment of it as a motor disorder.

There are occasions when patients with ulcerative colitis do need analgesics to relieve their abdominal pain. Acetaminophen (paracetamol, Tylenol) and propoxyphene (Darvon, Distalgesic) can be tried but are unlikely to help visceral pain. Stronger analgesics such as pentazocine (Talwin, Fortral) and meperidine (pethidine, Demerol) may be needed and can be prescribed with care. Opiates and their derivatives (including pentazocine and meperidine) and anticholingergics have a tendency to cause toxic dilatation of the colon in patients with acute ulcerative colitis.

A patient with ulcerative colitis who is suffering from pain due to conditions other than the colitis can be treated with analgesics in the same way as any other patient, except for the additional care that must be exercised when using the opiates (including codeine) in patients with active colitis.

PREVENTION OF AGGRAVATING FACTORS

There are a number of factors that appear to induce or exacerbate attacks of ulcerative colitis. These can be classified as diet, drugs, infections, psychological factors, and pregnancy. A number of patients have their first diagnosed attack of ulcerative colitis as a result of one or another of these. The disease usually then progresses largely independently of the aggravating factor.

Diet

Truelove (22) observed that a certain number of patients with ulcerative colitis, mainly younger patients, improved when placed on a milk-free diet and relapsed when milk was reintroduced. Attempts to demonstrate allergic reactions to milk protein in patients with ulcerative colitis have been unsuccessful, despite the evidence for immunological factors in the etiology of ulcerative colitis. What has been shown is that patients with hypolactasia, although no more predisposed than normal persons to the development of ulcerative colitis, have more severe attacks when they do relapse (23).

The authors do not recommend the indiscriminate trial of milk-free diets in ulcerative colitis. If a patient has a clear symptomatic intolerance to milk or if hypolactasia is diagnosed, then a lactose-free diet should be prescribed. This means that the diet should then be free of butter and cheese and other uncooked milk products. This can be a difficult diet to follow, especially for children. The diagnosis of hypolactasia is made directly by enzyme analysis of a jejunal biopsy specimen (this is not often available), or indirectly by means of a lactose tolerance test. The latter test should be performed in patients whose colitis is resistant to steroids or to the withdrawal of steroids in order to identify those who are likely to benefit from a lactose-free diet.

Other dietary restrictions in ulcerative colitis have little scientific basis. Bland diets are widely prescribed in the United States. In active colitis, it is possible that abrasion aggravates the inflammation. This is the rationale for excluding indigestible foods such as fruit skins and seeds and nuts and also raw vegetables such as celery, carrots, and lettuce. A few patients report that their disease improves when they avoid these foods. It is difficult to know whether or not this is a placebo effect, but the restriction is a harmless measure, provided that a vitamin C supplement is taken. The bland diet also often forbids all fresh fruit. This will reduce the bulk of the motions, but that may not be a good idea; it may be better for the motor function of the bowel to supply some soft roughage, particularly when inflammation is only mild. Of course, if a patient gives a history of a particular food aggravating the symptoms of colitis, then that food should be avoided. Patients with severe colitis are often treated with a totally intravenous regimen for a few days; and the benefit resulting from this, if it is real, is more likely to be due to an overall reduction in the activity of the gastrocolic motor reflexes or to the withdrawal of an unidentified toxic dietary antigen than to the withdrawal of mechanical roughage. Nevertheless, it is probably wise to prescribe a mechanically soft diet for a few days after the intravenous regimen. Other aspects of the bland diet may also be helpful by virtue of their diminishing the stimulation of the gastrocolic reflex, which may be the reason why some patients have aggravation of their symptoms following the ingestion of gaseous drinks.

Drugs

A number of drugs can exacerbate ulcerative colitis. Opiates and their derivatives, including codeine and dihydrocodeine (sold in Britain as DF-118), and anticholinergic drugs such as propantheline bromide, can give rise to toxic dilatation of the colon in a patient with severe colitis. Oral iron preparations frequently aggravate the symptoms and possibly also the degree of inflammation in ulcerative colitis. Broad-spectrum oral antibiotics should be avoided because of their tendency to cause a relapse of the disease. This is especially true with oral antibiotics in the penicillin group, including ampicillin. One broad-spectrum antibiotic that the authors have not seen to cause a flare-up of the disease and that may even be beneficial is the trimethoprim-sulfamethoxazole combination (cotrimoxazole, Bactrim, Septra, or Septrin), and otolaryngologists are advised to use this rather than penicillin and erythromycin when treating upper respiratory tract infections in patients with ulcerative colitis. Estrogens and progestogens in the contraceptive pill have been known to exacerbate ulcerative colitis. This is analogous to the effects of pregnancy on ulcerative colitis (see Chapter 19).

Infections

It is not uncommon for the first attack of ulcerative colitis to follow what appears to be an episode of infectious diarrhea, which may also have affected others eating at the same places as the patient. For the diagnosis of the ulcerative colitis, an infectious cause must then be excluded. However, even when an organism is identified, the ulcerative colitis often proves to be real; and from the future course of the patient, one can only conclude that the infection was an incidental factor that somehow stimulated that particular relapse. Patients with known disease also often relapse following exposure to a bowel infection. Agents specifically responsible for such infections have not been distinguished from other enteropathic organisms. The earlier theory that some cases of ulcerative colitis are the outcome of bacillary dysentery, suggested after World War II, has proved to be unfounded. The mechanism of the aggravating effect may be similar to that of hypolactasia: in viral gastroenteritis, and probably also in travelers' diarrhea due to certain strains of *Escherichia coli,* the jejunal villi are stunted and there is a functional deficiency of the mucosal enzymes, including lactase. Giardiasis is another infection that can affect the jejunum and cause a functional hypolactasia.

As a practical matter, the authors advise patients with ulcerative colitis to avoid travel to unhygienic parts of the world where they are liable to pick up an infectious diarrhea. Patients returning from these areas with a flare-up of their disease and other patients whose exacerbations may be due to an organism should be checked for *Giardia lamblia*. Giardiasis can be treated with metronidazole, but otherwise there is no specific treatment for these infections. Nonabsorbable sulfonamides have been proposed as prophylaxis for travelers against toxigenic *Escherichia coli* (83). Patients with ulcerative colitis already taking sulfasalazine may be protected to some extent.

Psychological Factors

The role of emotional factors in the incidence of ulcerative colitis is hotly debated. Many physicians believe passionately that there is an emotional element; yet no good published studies have demonstrated this. Most physicians treating ulcerative colitis can remember individual patients in whose history there was a manifestly stressful emotional environment, usually a pattern of resistance by a child to an overprotective parent, or a particularly stressful event, such as the death of a family member. The child with ulcerative colitis does tend to be protected by the parents, which may lead to a false impression of this factor as being primary when it may just be secondary to the disease. Emotional factors have been clearly demonstrated in the irritable colon syndrome, with which ulcerative colitis is occasionally confused. There is one published study suggesting that ulcerative colitis is more common in persons with hypochondriacal and hysterical traits than in their less neurotic siblings (84), but again there was no certainty that the affected patients did not develop these characteristics as a consequence of their disease.

Despite the doubts from the above discussion, the physician treating ulcerative colitis should pay attention to emotional factors in his patients. Emotional upsets increase colonic motility, and this may impair the remission of an attack of colitis. The physician should, of course, be sympathetic and understanding. He should identify anxiety states and depressive states, which may be secondary to the illness or aggravated by steroids. These deserve treatment either by supportive psychotherapy by the physician, who may also prescribe mild tranquilizers or antidepressants, or with the assistance of a psychiatrist.

Stress: Recommendations for Rest

Stress can be considered as a psychological factor that can exacerbate ulcerative colitis. Mental stress is probably similar to other emotional factors in its effect on quiescent ulcerative colitis. It is likely (but not proved) that it can reactivate the colitis. In the patient with active disease, the avoidance of stress should be diligent. Patients with severe disease are normally hospitalized, and this environment should not be too hectic (as some large hospitals nowadays unfortunately are becoming). Rest in the hospital should help calm the patient from all his stresses and should assist healing. Patients with moderate disease should also be rested, to a certain extent, though they can remain mildly active rather than confined to bed or to other restrictive surroundings where they may become introverted. Bed rest as such should be avoided as much as possible in ulcerative colitis, and the patient should walk a short distance every hour or so to minimize the risk of venous thrombosis, which can occur in ulcerative colitis. Patients with mild colitis should remain at work but avoid excessive competition or long hours.

In a chronic disease such as ulcerative colitis, it is important to keep patients as occupied and productive as possible. This will contribute positively to their moods and attitudes. The same applies to these patients with regard to athletic activity. They can gently jog short distances, play friendly games of golf, or swim short distances, but they should not subject themselves to competitive stresses in their sports. Brisk walks of one or two miles are an appropriate activity.

Pregnancy

The management of patients with ulcerative colitis who become pregnant, including patients who develop their colitis for the first time during pregnancy, is discussed in Chapter 19. Pregnancy is a definite aggravating factor in ulcerative colitis. About one-third of patients with inactive disease and about two-thirds with active disease have exacerbation either during pregnancy or immediately postpartum. There are many patients who have their first diagnosed attack of ulcerative colitis during or immediately after a pregnancy.

Unwanted pregnancy should therefore be avoided in patients with ulcerative colitis. Those with moderately active disease should be told that they should not become pregnant at least until a remission is induced. Oral contraceptives containing estrogens and progestogens are not an ideal mode of preventing pregnancy in patients with ulcerative colitis, because the hormonal patterns induced are similar to those of pregnancy; but the incidence of flare-ups of the disease associated with the use of these contraceptives is not as great as that related to pregnancy itself. If the patient can successfully avoid pregnancy by other means of contraception, that is to be preferred; but it is better to use the oral contraceptives than to risk an unintentional pregnancy.

CONCLUSION

From the above discussion, it will be apparent that there is more to the medical management of ulcerative colitis than simply the prescription of steroids and sulfasalazine, important though these drugs are.

14

TREATMENT OF COMPLICATIONS

COLONIC COMPLICATIONS

The colorectal complications of ulcerative colitis are mostly dealt with surgically, and their surgical management will be described in Chapter 16. They include perforation, abscess formation, peritonitis, and carcinoma of the colon. The complications of hemorrhage and acute dilatation of the colon can be considered as indicators of particularly severe primary disease and are not necessarily treated surgically if they respond rapidly to medical management. Cancer of the colon complicating ulcerative colitis is an absolute indication for early surgery.

Polyps

The treatment of adenomatous polyps arising in the colon of a patient with ulcerative colitis is to remove them colonoscopically. Colotomy in a patient with ulcerative colitis which is at all active is a dangerous procedure, but it can be done if the colitis is quiescent; however, colonoscopy is usually easier in patients with ulcerative colitis than in normal persons because of the shortening of the colon. Inflammatory pseudopolyps do not warrant removal (except for diagnosis when their nature is in doubt); nor do they require any treatment *per se.*

Strictures

Strictures of the colon do not need treatment provided one is assured that they are benign (either by colonoscopic biopsy and cytology or, if colonoscopy is not possible, from definite radiological signs of their benign nature). Nonmalignant strictures of the colon should not cause significant problems to the patient. The presence of a malignant stricture is an indication for total colectomy.

PERIANAL COMPLICATIONS

Perianal complications are less common in ulcerative colitis than in Crohn's disease. In fact, the presence of anal fissures or fistulas should raise the possibility of a diagnosis of Crohn's disease rather than ulcerative colitis. Anal lesions in inflammatory bowel disease should be dealt with as conservatively as possible, since surgical interference may lead to further perianal troubles. Pruritus ani and uncomfortable anal lesions should be treated with local ointments, creams, or suppositories containing a barrier compound (such as zinc oxide), a local anesthetic, and hydrocortisone. An antibiotic, frequently neomycin in proprietary preparations, is not indicated and often sensitizes the anal skin, which can then become the site of a dermatitis. Proprietary preparations in the United States include Anusol-HC (barrier compounds plus hydrocortisone) and Nupercainal (dibucaine—a local anesthetic—plus zinc oxide), these being available as creams or suppositories. A recent study has shown that the surgical management of hemorrhoids is fairly free from complications in patients with ulcerative colitis (unlike the situation in Crohn's disease) (85).

EXTRAINTESTINAL COMPLICATIONS

The presence of extraintestinal complications of ulcerative colitis has a bearing on the management of the primary bowel disease. All the extraintestinal manifestations have a tendency to worsen as the colitis flares up and to improve as the colitis is successfully treated; but this is not invariably the case. The liver disease and ankylosing spondylitis can progress following total colectomy, whereas the other systemic complications all remit when the colon is removed. Thus, the presence of these complications may increase the urgency of dealing with the bowel disease, indicating more vigorous medical therapy, usually in the form of larger doses of steroids; and sometimes the complications result in an earlier decision to proceed to surgery.

Arthritis

The arthritis associated with ulcerative colitis is treated specifically by short courses of corticosteroids, which will also help to suppress the colitis. Most patients respond. Salicylates can be used, rather than steroids, when the arthritis is only mild. Crippling arthritis which is resistant to steroid therapy, and for which other anti-inflammatory agents, such as phenylbutazone and indomethacin, have been tried, may very occasionally be an indication for colectomy. One must be sure that the arthritis really is the arthritis of ulcerative colitis (which can be difficult), but the ulcerative colitis itself must be of some degree of activity. Even if the arthritis is then really of the rheumatoid arthritis type, the removal of a colon with active ulcerative colitis often leads to improvement of the arthritis.

Sacroiliitis

Inflammation of the sacroiliac joints occurring in association with ulcerative colitis is treated by suppression of the bowel disease with steroids, which also help the sacroiliitis. Other analgesics, particularly of the anti-inflammatory group, may be needed.

Ankylosing Spondylitis

When ankylosing spondylitis occurs in association with ulcerative colitis, it generally progresses independently of the colitis; but there can be some improvement as the colitis is successfully treated. The treatment of the spondylitis is with analgesics, particularly those with an anti-inflammatory action, such as aspirin and phenylbutazone. Total colectomy does not cure and often does not prevent progression of ankylosing spondylitis.

Skin Complications

Pyoderma gangrenosum is the most dangerous of the skin complications of ulcerative colitis; and the activity of the bowel disease should be promptly suppressed with as much steroid as is required. If the colitis is resistant to steroid therapy, then a severe pyoderma is an indication for colectomy. Azathioprine should never be used in a patient with pyoderma gangrenosum because of the risk of a complicating bacterial skin infection.

Erythema nodosum remits as the colitis remits. The condition is a sign that there is some disease activity in the bowel, but it is not a complication that gives a great deal of trouble in itself. In a patient taking sulfasalazine or other sulfonamides, erythema nodosum is occasionally due to the drug, and withdrawal of the sulfonamide may help it to remit.

Oral Aphthous Ulcers

Oral aphthous ulcers frequently occur in patients with ulcerative colitis. In the main, they cause little trouble. Betamethasone valereate pellets can be sucked against the ulcers. More extensive aphthous ulceration can be treated with mouthwashes of hydrocortisone, 100 mg dissolved in a glass of warm water each day, with a quarter of the solution being used as a mouthwash after each meal. In Britain, carbenoxolone sodium pellets (Bioral) are available and have been found to accelerate the healing of oral aphthous ulcers.

Ocular Complications

Ocular complications respond to treatment of the colitis: the presence of iritis or episcleritis is an indication for oral steroid therapy. Patients with conjunctivitis associated with ulcerative colitis can use prednisolone drops in the eyes if the colonic disease does not warrant a sufficiently effective dose of oral steroids. In that instance one must be sure that there is not an infectious conjunctivitis. One clue in ulcerative colitis is that the condition is usually bilateral. Iritis generally requires the use of local steroid eye drops and a powerful local miotic agent, but this condition must be managed in cooperation with an ophthalmologist.

Liver Disease

Most of the hepatobiliary complications of ulcerative colitis can remit if the colitis itself is treated (86). This may require a colectomy. Sclerosing cholangitis and chronic hepatitis frequently progress despite suppression of the colitis and despite removal of the diseased bowel; and established cirrhosis is a permanent situation. Antibiotics have not been shown to help the pericholangitis associated with ulcerative colitis, although if a patient with pericholangitis has a fever, it is best to cover a possible bacterial infection with an antibiotic, the current recommendation for cholangitis associated with gallstones being gentamicin. Ampicillin is less toxic and is probably indicated in mild feverish cases. Sclerosing cholangitis that is causing obstruction of the biliary tree can be treated in some cases by drainage of a dilated biliary radicle in the liver through a Rodney Smith tube into the duodenum, with the tube passing through a loop of ileum which is brought up into the right upper quadrant.

The fatty liver that is frequent in ulcerative colitis should remit when nutrition is restored and the acute disease is treated.

Chronic active hepatitis, if transaminases are significantly affected or the patient is jaundiced or symptomatic from the liver disease, and if this diagnosis is confirmed on liver biopsy, is treated with either prednisone, 20 mg daily, or prednisone, 10 mg daily, plus azathioprine, 50 to 100 mg daily, for several months or until the serum transaminase levels improve (87). It can be seen that the same course of medications can be used to treat both the liver disease and the ulcerative colitis.

Patients with hepatic complications of ulcerative colitis should probably abstain from taking alcohol.

Biliary Tract Carcinoma

Radical surgical removal can be attempted as a cure of biliary tract carcinoma, but this condition has been uniformly fatal, despite treatment, whenever it has been diagnosed (39). Relief of pruritus due to biliary obstruction may be an indication for a palliative resection or a bypass procedure for the bile flow (e.g., a choledochojejunostomy).

Gallstones

Although gallstones are not a specific complication of ulcerative colitis, a few points can be made concerning the management of gallstones occurring in patients with ulcerative colitis. In fit patients, gallstones are considered to be an indication for cholecystectomy; but in patients with ulcerative colitis that is active or is requiring steroids for control, the presence of asymptomatic gallstones should not be an indication for surgery on the gallbladder. When the colitis has become quiescent and systemic steroids are no longer being used, the removal of a calculous gallbladder by a skillful surgeon is a wise move and will remove one possible cause of hepatobiliary disease and may simplify the differential diagnosis of biliary obstruction should that develop at a later stage.

Thromboembolic Disorders

When venous thrombosis and pulmonary embolism occur in patients with ulcerative colitis, the use of anticoagulants is restricted by the danger of hemorrhage from the inflamed colon, which may already be bleeding. The risks of the thrombosis or embolism must be carefully weighed against the risks of treatment. When leg vein thrombosis is superficial, anticoagulants should not be used in ulcerative colitis (and they should probably not be used in otherwise normal patients). The legs should be bandaged tightly, and aspirin should be given. When there is deep vein thrombosis, anticoagulants should be given if the patient is not bleeding from the colon, but withheld if there is active bleeding. Aspirin may be beneficial in the latter situation.

If anticoagulation is to be instituted, heparin may be preferable to coumarins because its anticoagulant effect is rapidly reversed by protamine and its lytic effect on venous thrombi may be greater than that of the coumarins. On the other hand, some surgeons find that patients given heparin bleed more easily during surgery than patients given coumarin. Patients who have recently bled or patients whose colitis may be expected to have a high probability of bleeding should be treated with lose-dose heparin, 5,000 units every 12 hours in an intravenous infusion. At the same time, the colitis must be suppressed with as much prednisone as may be required.

The difficulty arises when pulmonary emboli occur in a patient who is bleeding from ulcerative colitis. The only course of action one can take is to prevent the thrombi from reaching the heart and lungs by inserting an "umbrella" catheter into the inferior vena cava, or by plication of the vena cava, which can be done at the colectomy operation.

Renal Calculi

The hyperoxaluria that develops in various intestinal diseases is believed to be related to ileal dysfunction, which therefore cannot be implicated in patients with ulcerative colitis rather than Crohn's disease. There must be other mechanisms responsible for the increased incidence of phosphate, oxalate, and uric acid stones in patients with ulcerative colitis. The best one can do in prophylaxis is to keep patients with ulcerative colitis well hydrated, especially in hot weather and following physical exertion; to minimize the use of corticosteroids; to alkalinize the urine with bicarbonate if patients are found to have uric acid stones or uric acid crystals in the urine; and to restrict dietary oxalates in those who have oxalate crystals on urine analysis. Nuts, mushrooms, chocolate, and rhubarb are foods that contain significant amounts of oxalates and are to be avoided if hyperoxaluria is detected. Avoidance of purine-containing foods that is sufficiently rigorous to diminish uric acid in the urine is extremely difficult. Urinary alkalinization and treatment of hyperuricemia with allopurinol are more effective ways of preventing uric acid stones. Suppression of activity of the colitis can be presumed to be helpful in preventing the formation of all forms of urinary calculi, but steroids used on a long-term basis probably aggravate the tendency to the formation of calculi.

Once urinary calculi have been diagnosed, they are treated no differently than in patients who do not have ulcerative colitis: a high fluid intake is in order and, if necessary, retrograde catheterization of the ureters and surgical removal of the calculi. The urine must be checked frequently for infections that may need to be treated.

Although suppression of the colitis is theoretically helpful in preventing and treating urinary calculi, the use of steroids can be counterproductive and the surgical removal of the colon leaves an ileostomy that results in an even greater tendency to stone formation, as a result of the tendency to dehydration in ileostomy patients.

Anemia, Dehydration, Malnutrition

The management of these complications, which are merely secondary to the colonic pathology, was covered in the previous chapter.

Other Extracolonic Manifestations of Ulcerative Colitis

In treating the extracolonic associations that appear to be of immunological origin, such as carditis, the principles are to treat with corticosteroids and to suppress the colitis as much as possible.

15

FOLLOW-UP

Patients with ulcerative colitis who are symptomatic generally consult their physicians, and their disease can then be diagnosed and treated. Once a patient is known to have ulcerative colitis, there should be a regular schedule to visit the specialist, whether or not the disease is troublesome and regardless of how many years there has been freedom from symptoms.

THE IMPORTANCE OF REGULAR VISITS

The reasons for regular follow-up of patients with ulcerative colitis can be listed and should be stressed to patients:

1. Many physicians believe in an annual checkup for the apparently healthy person. The necessity for this is sometimes debated, but in patients with ulcerative colitis there are many associated and secondary conditions that are prone to occur even if the patient is asymptomatic, conditions such as renal stones and hepatobiliary disorders (Chapter 8), which are important to detect and treat early.

2. The outcome of an attack of ulcerative colitis will be more favorable if it is treated sooner rather than later. It is better to treat before the patient has become anemic, malnourished, or hypovolemic. Since attacks of colitis usually build up over a few days, a planned checkup will not usually occur at the ideal moment for treatment that could prevent progression to severity; therefore, the patient must be encouraged to call the physician as soon as the earliest symptoms occur. Mildly active disease can be detected at a follow-up visit, whereas even moderately active disease is often ignored by the patient. Suppression of the inflammation at an early stage by appropriate medication can prevent the progression to a serious attack. Also, the risk of carcinoma of the colon developing in patients with long-standing cases of ulcerative colitis is greater the more active the disease has been. One can possibly conclude from this that better suppression of the inflammatory activity lessens the carcinogenic risk.

3. Specific aggravating factors can be dealt with by the physician before they exacerbate an attack of the disease. Social and emotional problems can be discussed, to avoid the development of undue stress. Medications that may be prescribed by other specialists, and that may upset the bowel (e.g., antibiotics, iron), can be reviewed.

4. Many asymptomatic patients still require medication. In most cases this will be sulfasalazine. The side effects of sulfasalazine include anemia and other blood dyscrasias, and the patient taking sulfasalazine should have regular appointments with his physician so that regular blood counts can be done and the effects of the drug can be monitored.

5. Once the patient has had ulcerative colitis for seven years or more (and this includes years prior to the diagnosis of the disease in which typical symptoms can be recalled), there is an increased tendency for carcinoma of the colon to develop. The risk increases with the length and severity of the history of the ulcerative colitis and is greater the younger the age of onset. The tumors that develop are more often intramucosal and less often polypoid than in noncolitics, and this, together with the fact that the barium enema X-ray appearances are usually abnormal in ulcerative colitis even without complicating carcinoma, makes the diagnosis of cancer more difficult than is normally the case. There are means of early diagnosis of cancer of the colon in patients with ulcerative colitis, which will be discussed later in this chapter, and they require regular visits by the patient to the physician's office or clinic.

6. The knowledge of the potential dangers of having ulcerative colitis can cause anxiety in the patient. A regular visit to the physician can be used to reassure the patient of the inactivity of the condition.

A Primary Physician

In countries where there is no established tradition of a primary physician (as there is in Great Britain), it is important that the patient with ulcerative colitis identify a primary physician with whom all other specialists should communicate. This may be a family practitioner, a general internist, or a gastroenterologist, so long as the physician is aware of the multisystem nature of ulcerative colitis and of its complications. It may be that a patient will see an ophthalmologist for treatment of uveitis that is complicating his ulcerative colitis, but the eye specialist is not aware that the patient has had colitis, any more than the physician treating the colitis is aware that the patient is seeing an ophthalmologist.

FOLLOW-UP OBSERVATIONS

As a general rule, the authors would recommend that the patient in whom ulcerative colitis has once been diagnosed (including cases of ulcerative proctitis limited to the rectum) should see a physician with experience in gastroenterology at least once every six months. The patient should be questioned about symptoms of the disease, including stool form and frequency, the presence or absence of blood, and the experience of abdominal or rectal pain. The weight should be recorded at each visit. For the patient who is having normal bowel movements without blood and with no other symptoms and who has not yet had the disease for seven years, a sigmoidoscopy need only be performed annually. If there is any question at all about disease activity at a particular time, then a sigmoidoscopy should be done at that time. A blood count (hemoglobin, hematocrit, red cell indexes, and white cell count) should be performed annually if the patient is not taking sulfasalazine, but more frequently, say every three months, if the patient is taking that drug; in patients taking azathioprine, these values need to be determined every three weeks or so, together with a platelet count. A multichannel biochemical screen is worth doing once a year in order to detect rises in blood urea and alkaline phosphatase and transaminases (pointing to liver disease associated with the colitis) and lowering of the serum albumin. Urinalysis should also be performed at least once a year to look for infection and for crystals and red blood cells indicating the formation of calculi.

EARLY DETECTION OF COLONIC CARCINOMA

For patients who have had ulcerative colitis for seven years or more, a more diligent follow-up program is advised. Unfortunately, even the idealistic perfection of a monthly colonoscopy (were this feasible, which it is not) would probably not detect all carcinomas at an operable stage. The authors have had experience, and there have been reports in the literature, of colitic patients with negative colonoscopies who turned out to have a carcinoma. Indicators and procedures in investigating suspicion of carcinoma comprise the following:

1. *Symptoms:* These include a change in bowel habit, rectal bleeding, and abdominal and rectal pain. The symptoms of a carcinoma cannot really be distinguished from those of a flare-up of ulcerative colitis, so that any suggestion of a flare-up, however mild, in a patient with seven or more years of ulcerative colitis must be regarded as a potential indicator of a carcinoma.
2. *Blood count:* The development of anemia or of a leukocytosis or a rise in the erythrocyte sedimentation rate in a patient who is otherwise well should raise the suspicion of a carcinoma.
3. *Sigmoidoscopy:* If a tumor is within reach of the sigmoidoscope, it should be detectable at sigmoidoscopy. The examination is sometimes limited by discomfort in the patient or by lack of skill in the examiner, and examinations have been reported as negative when a tumor has been present. The rigid sigmoidoscope cannot detect lesions above 30 cm (although the new flexible fiberoptic sigmoidoscope reaches 60 cm—see Chapter 11); and the carcinomas that occur in ulcerative colitis are less likely to be in the rectosigmoid than carcinoma of the colon in noncolitics.
4. *Colonoscopy:* A good colonoscopist can usually, but by no means always, perform a complete endoscopic examination of the colon in a patient with ulcerative colitis. In most cases this will detect a carcinoma if one is present. The frequency with which this study can be performed is limited by the time required (which is translated into its high cost) and the discomfort in the patient. The procedure has a very small, but measurable, risk.
5. *Barium enema X-ray (air-contrast) examination:* This study, which is more convenient to perform than colonsocopy, can detect carcinoma in many cases, though it is by no means infallible. The benign strictures that occur in patients with ulcerative colitis complicate the radiological reading and diminish the accuracy with which carcinoma can be diagnosed. If the colitis is of moderate or

severe activity, the air-contrast examination carries a greater risk of exacerbating the disease than a conventional barium enema X-ray examination, and only the latter should be performed.

6. *Detection of precancer on biopsy:* The presence of epithelial dysplasia as an index of the presence of occult carcinoma or a premalignant tendency was discussed in Chapter 4. From experience reported in the literature and from the authors' own experience, between one-quarter and one-half of patients with histological evidence of epithelial dysplasia (see Figure 4–6) in a nonregenerating, noninflamed mucosa in long-standing ulcerative colitis will prove to have a carcinoma if total colectomy is performed. Morson and Pang (88), who first described this premalignant lesion, found that it was fairly diffuse in the colon.

The more biopsy specimens that are taken, the greater the likelihood that the lesion will be found, but the return to the patient for each additional biopsy after the first is not very great. If colonoscopy is being performed for any reason in a patient with long-standing ulcerative colitis, then at least six biopsy specimens from different parts of the colon should be screened for dysplastic change; but there is a good pick-up rate from rectal biopsy alone through the sigmoidoscope.

7. *Detection of elevated levels of serum carcinoembryonic antigen (CEA):* The CEA level is elevated in the majority of patients with carcinoma of the colon, whether or not there is ulcerative colitis. The value of this measurement in detecting carcinoma in patients who have ulcerative colitis is severely limited by the fact that one-third of patients with ulcerative colitis have elevated CEA levels whether or not they have a carcinoma. The discrimination of colitic patients who have carcinoma or precancer by measurement of serum CEA is almost impossible. The one instance in which it may help is if the CEA level is very high, say, above 40 ng per ml. In one series, one-quarter of patients with cancer or precancer complicating ulcerative colitis had such high CEA levels, whereas none of 140 patients without cancer or precancer had such a high level (89). A recent report has indicated that detection of CEA in the *tissue* of rectal biopsy specimens in ulcerative colitis may be an index of premalignant change (90); and this may prove to be of more help than the serum CEA measurement.

The authors' recommendation for follow-up of patients with more than seven years of ulcerative colitis is to perform a blood count and sigmoidoscopy at the six-monthly visit. One or two rectal biopsy specimens should be taken at the sigmoidoscopy, on the posterior wall at 10 cm, which is below the peritoneal reflection. An air-contrast barium enema X-ray examination should be performed annually. The authors cannot yet firmly recommend regular colonoscopy as part of the follow-up of the asymptomatic patient, but a suspicious flare-up of symptoms or a doubtful appearance on the barium enema X-ray film can be an indication for colonoscopy with multiple biopsies in the search for cancer or precancer.

16

SURGICAL TREATMENT

The standard surgical operation used in the treatment of ulcerative colitis is total proctocolectomy with a permanent ileostomy. This operation cures the colonic disease and leads to a remission or improvement in most of the peripheral manifestations of ulcerative colitis. This discussion will initially confine itself to this particular operation. Later in the chapter, other surgical procedures that are used to treat the primary disease will be mentioned.

INDICATIONS FOR COLECTOMY

Absolute Indications

Perforation

Evidence of or suspicion of colonic perforation in ulcerative colitis is an absolute indication for a colectomy. If there is free perforation and peritonitis, the colectomy must be performed as an emergency.

Abscess Formation

If the perforation has resulted in abscess formation without peritonitis, then a few hours or days can be spent in improving the general condition of the patient, by the correction of dehydration, hypoalbuminemia, or anemia, or by the use of antibiotic therapy.

Colonic Carcinoma

The occurrence of a colonic carcinoma complicating ulcerative colitis is an absolute indication for total colectomy, both as treatment of the tumor and as prevention of further carcinomas developing (unless the malignancy is disseminated and the patient is cachectic). Colonic carcinomas complicating ulcerative colitis are often multiple; and, in this premalignant disease, once one tumor has appeared, then there is considerable potential for further carcinogenesis.

Relative Indications

Failure of Medical Management

The point at which medical management can be said to have failed requires careful judgment, and the criteria for such a decision have been discussed in Chapter 13. As stated in that chapter, this is probably the most usual indication for colectomy.

Massive Hemorrhage

Hemorrhage uncontrollable by transfusion and other medical measures is really a failure of medical management, but it is not infrequently an indication in itself for an urgent or semi-urgent colectomy.

Toxic Dilatation of the Colon

If toxic dilatation of the colon persists, medical management can be considered to have failed. Some physicians regard the presence of toxic dilatation as an absolute indication for colectomy. The authors regard gross dilatation (as judged clinically and on plain abdominal X-ray) as an absolute indication, but lesser degrees of dilatation are frequent. When toxic dilatation has persisted for more than 48 hours, the results of surgery are much worse than if colectomy is done within the first 48 hours (91). In skilled hands, medical management can be tried for up to 48 hours, with close observation of the patient; but any signs of increase in the dilatation or persistence beyond 24 to 48 hours must be regarded as an indication for immediate colectomy.

Peripheral Manifestations of Ulcerative Colitis

The presence and severity of peripheral manifestations of ulcerative colitis are sometimes an indication for colectomy, as discussed in Chapter 14.

Epithelial Dysplasia

The changes of moderate or severe epithelial dysplasia seen in rectal or colonoscopic biopsy specimens are an indication that there is a considerable likelihood of the development, or even of the presence, of colonic carcinoma complicating the colitis (Chapter 4). The authors regard moderate or severe dysplasia in a patient with ulcerative colitis of more than seven years' duration as an indication for colectomy (except in the old and frail), although this is still a controversial point.

Strictures

The presence of a malignant or possibly malignant stricture is an indication for total colectomy. Benign strictures rarely cause any ill effects. If, unusually, they do cause obstruction to the flow of stool, a partial colectomy can be performed if the ulcerative colitis is quiescent. If the colitis is active, a total colectomy may be needed. This may be an indication for an ileorectal anastomosis (see below).

Multiple Indications

There are five relative indications for colectomy which can summate with each other in a decision for colectomy. They are as follows: persistence of symptoms of colitis (pain and diarrhea); continuing blood loss; refractory or progressive peripheral manifestations of ulcerative colitis; certain pointers of a particular predisposition to develop carcinoma (long history, young age of onset, chronic disease activity); and the presence of mild epithelial dysplasia seen in biopsy specimens.

PROCTOCOLECTOMY WITH AN ILEOSTOMY

This book will not attempt to describe surgical techniques in detail, but there are some points that are of relevance to the internist who is considering referring a patient for surgery. The operation of panproctocolectomy involves the removal of the entire large bowel, from the ileum close to the ileocecal valve down to and including the rectum. A combined abdominal and perineal approach is used, and two surgeons can operate together. For the abdominal incision, some surgeons use a left paramedian longitudinal incision, whereas others prefer a transverse subumbilical incision.

Perimuscular Excision of the Rectum

Perimuscular excision of the rectum is the technique recommended by Lee and Dowling of Oxford, England (92). In the rectum, the surgeon works as closely as possible to the muscle wall, using local infusions of norepinephrine (1: 200,000) to make a bloodless field in order to make this close dissection in the perimuscular space. The anterior and posterior walls of the rectum are dissected free, prior to careful dissection of the lateral walls. This is in order not to disturb the parasympathetic nerve plexus to the genitalia and the urethra. These nerves run in the presacral fat pad immediately lateral to the rectum. If this technique is used, 90 to 95% of men should retain normal sexual function. The operating time is increased; so the presence of two surgeons working together will speed up the operation. It may not be possible to perform perimuscular excision at an emergency operation, so that a subtotal colectomy with a temporary rectomucous fistula may be the operation of choice in this situation (see below).

Ulcerative Colitis Complicated by Carcinoma

The dissection close to the wall of the rectum is not appropriate when there is cancer in the rectosigmoid. In that case, a wide excision is required, including the pelvic lymph nodes. If the cancer is confined to the proximal descending colon or is more proximal to that, or if there are only premalignant changes rather than actual cancer, then a perimuscular excision can still be done. The wide excision used in cancer almost inevitably damages the nervi erigentes and interferes with sexual function in the male.

The Construction of the Ileostomy

The Site

The ileostomy should be placed on the anterior abdominal wall in the right lower quadrant (Figure 16–1). It should be low enough for the patient to wear the belt of the ileostomy bag around the waist, high enough for a reasonably sized bag to hand mostly in the right iliac fossa (see Figure 17–1), medial to the anterior superior iliac spine so that the flange of the ileostomy appliance does not impinge on the iliac crest, and lateral to the umbilicus so that the ileostomy flange is clear of the umbilicus.

Fashioning the Ileostomy

The Brooke technique (93) is now the standard for the ileostomy, since it obviates many of the problems encountered with earlier methods. The ileal mucosa

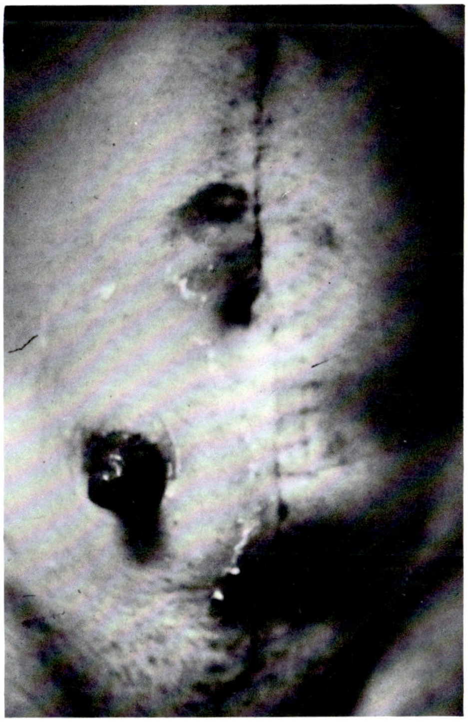

FIGURE 16–1
Recently constructed ileostomy in its optimum site.

is everted over the ileum, which should protrude about 2 cm from the abdomen. The ileal mucosa is then stitched to the abdominal wall.

Care of the ileostomy and details of ileostomy appliances are discussed in Chapter 17.

PREOPERATIVE AND POSTOPERATIVE CARE

Preoperative Care

The time available for preoperative preparation for colectomy naturally depends on the urgency of the procedure. In an emergency situation, there is no time for preoperative preparation. In a semi-urgent situation, there may be time to correct any deficits in the hemoglobin level, the plasma albumin level, and the serum potassium. For a non-urgent colectomy, these factors should be restored to normal if any of them is abnormal. Clotting parameters should also be checked, and routine preoperative electrocardiograms and pulmonary function tests are usually requested for the anesthesiologist. Preoperative deep breathing exercises should be a routine.

Preoperative hyperalimentation is recommended in some circles for nutritionally depleted patients about to undergo proctocolectomy. In general, the authors believe that the source of the protein loss, namely the colon, should be removed as soon as possible; but they are in favor of two to four weeks of preoperative hyperalimentation in severely underweight patients with *mild* or *mild-to-moderate* activity of their ulcerative colitis seen on sigmoidoscopic or colonoscopic examination. The amateur should not engage in the use of parenteral hyperalimentation because of grave dangers of infection, which are particularly common when a hospital does not have a hyperalimentation team (94).

A patient with active colitis will normally not need any bowel preparation because the bloody diarrhea will already have cleared the colon of feces. Patients with quiescent colitis who come to colectomy (most often because of cancer or a high cancer risk) can be given magnesium sulfate twice daily for three days preoperatively, and they can be given gentle tapwater enemas if there is no proctitis. All patients should be restricted to clear liquids for four or five days before the operation.

Antibiotics should not be part of routine preoperative preparation in patients with ulcerative colitis. Broad-spectrum antibiotics can cause the disease to flare up in the hours preceding the surgery. However, when there has been sepsis or perforation, kanamycin sulfate capsules (Kantrex, Bristol Laboratories) can be given for 48 hours preoperatively. The dosage is 1 gm hourly for four hours and then 1 gm six-hourly until the surgery.

A nasogastric tube is introduced shortly after the premedication for the operation.

Psychological preparation of the patient for the ileostomy is important. An ileostomy patient of the same sex and similar age and social background can meet the patient before the operation in order to provide reassurance that a reasonably normal life can be compatible with an ileostomy.

Postoperative Management

Following the operation, the patient should be kept under close observation in a recovery ward for four hours or so, before returning him to his room. To reduce the danger of the development of deep venous thrombosis, the patient should be encouraged to get up out of bed on the day of surgery. Postoperative physical therapy in the form of deep breathing exercises and leg exercises should be emphasized.

As far as postoperative feeding is concerned, the progression to full feeding should be rather cautious. Intravenous alimentation and nasogastric suction should be continued until bowel sounds are audible with the stethoscope and the ileostomy is seen to put out fluid. The nasogastric tube should then be removed, and 24 hours later, water should be given to drink. The patient should be observed carefully for signs of gastric dilatation, and if this does develop, the nasogastric tube should be reinserted and oral drinks should be withheld for at least another 48 hours. If drinks of water are tolerated satisfactorily, clear liquids in increasing amounts should be given over the next three days. Following that, for three further days, increasing amounts of liquidized foods should be given, and then a soft diet for three days, before introducing solid foods, which must be chewed well.

Many patients feel that they must eat normal food as soon as possible to prove that they have been cured of their ulcerative colitis and that they now have "normal" bowel function. They should be told that a few more days of patience will be well rewarded in a smoother postoperative course.

Preoperative and Postoperative Steroids

Patients with ulcerative colitis who have received no oral steroids and not more than three steroid enemas weekly in the preceding six months require no steroid supplementation at the time of colectomy. Patients who have received steroids in the previous six months but who are not taking steroids at the time of the operation should be given 100 mg of hydrocortisone intramuscularly with the premedication for surgery and then 100 mg six-hourly for 72 hours after the operation. The dose of hydrocortisone can then be progressively halved each day subsequently.

Patients who are receiving steroids at the time of surgery can also be treated with 100 mg of hydrocortisone six-hourly for 72 hours after surgery. The steroids should then be tailed off a little more slowly, giving, say, 300 mg of hydrocortisone on the fourth postoperative day, and then 250 mg, 200 mg, 150 mg, 100 mg, 75 mg, 50 mg, and 25 mg on successive days.

THE COMPLICATIONS OF PROCTOCOLECTOMY

The overall death rate from protocolectomy is about 5%, although the age of the patient, the severity of his illness, the urgency of the surgery, and the experience of the surgeon influence the complication rate and the death rate. Roughly two-thirds of palients have no significant postoperative complications. Ten to twenty percent will be detained in the hospital as a result of postoperative complications; and between 5 and 15% will need readmission because of complications, usually related to the ileostomy.

Hemorrhage

After a total colectomy, many blood vessels will have been tied, and the patient should be watched diligently for postoperative hemorrhage.

The Abdominal Wound

Any abdominal wound can become infected or can rupture. In ulcerative colitis, severe inflammation in the resected colon increases the likelihood of postoperative infective complications, both in the wound and more generally in the abdomen. Preoperative steroids have frequently been used in treating ulcerative colitis, and they predispose to postoperative infection and to poor wound healing.

With an infected wound, closure will be delayed and should be allowed to be secondary. Wound abscesses should be sought by gloved digital probing, and they should be drained if present. Pus in wounds should be cultured, but antibiotics should be used only if there is spreading cellulitis or if there is evidence of more generalized infection. Otherwise, the wound should be irrigated two or three times daily with sterile saline. A ruptured wound can be resutured when clean. An incisional hernia is a postoperative complication related to the abdominal wound.

The Perineal Wound

Slow healing of the perineal wound is very common, and complete healing may take months or even years. The patient should be warned preoperatively that this may happen. Slow healing is more common in women than in men. Primary closure of this wound with a small drain, rather than packing, minimizes the likelihood of slow healing. If healing of this wound is delayed, secondary suture should not be performed. Saline irrigation once or twice daily is indicated, and the patient should wear a clean perineal pad. Eventually, nearly all perineal wounds do close.

Intra-Abdominal Infection

When proctocolectomy is an emergency operation in patients with ulcerative colitis, fecal soiling of the peritoneum is common. Such soiling may occur even in elective operations. Postoperative peritonitis and intra-abdominal abscesses, in the pelvis and in the subphrenic areas, are not infrequent and can be fatal. Peritonitis may be difficult to detect in the patient who has been receiving steroids. Fever may be suppressed, but tachycardia is a clue. Postoperative ileus for more than about five days in a patient who does not appear to be completely well may also be an indication that there is peritonitis. If peritonitis is suspected, a broad-spectrum antibiotic combination that covers both aerobes and anaerobes should be prescribed, gentamicin with clindamycin being suitable. (There is no risk of membranous colitis following total colectomy.) Consideration should be given to reexploration of the abdomen. There may be strangulation or perforation or ischemia of the remaining small bowel.

A pelvic abscess is treated by perineal drainage. A subphrenic abscess is treated initially with broad-spectrum antibiotics, but it may need drainage through the bed of the twelfth rib.

Intestinal Obstruction

It is surprising to note that intestinal obstruction is one of the commonest factors leading to death following proctocolectomy. Adhesions are the usual initiating factor. Internal hernias, for instance into the lateral space, are also causes of obstruction, and obstruction can occur in relation to the ileostomy. The complication of intestinal obstruction can occur early or later postoperatively (years afterwards). Awareness of this possible development will result in earlier detection and earlier and safer treatment.

Ileostomy Complications

Between 10 and 20% of patients with an ileostomy following proctocolectomy for ulcerative colitis will require some form of surgical revision of the stoma. The ileostomy may be too tight; it may prolapse; a fistula may form next to the stoma; or a para-ileostomy hernia may develop. Ileostomy obstruction and para-ileostomy hernia are causes of intestinal obstruction.

Ileostomy dysfunction and peristomal dermatitis are complications that are discussed in Chapter 17.

Prestomal Ileitis

There is a dispute as to the existence of prestomal ileitis in patients who have had proctocolectomy for ulcerative colitis. The accepted view, to which the authors subscribe, is that usually the occurrence of prestomal ileitis is an indication that the patient was really suffering from Crohn's colitis and reexamination of pathological material from the colectomy specimen usually confirms this. However, this may not be a golden rule, and there seem to be patients who certainly had had ulcerative colitis and then develop prestomal ileitis, but not a large number.

Urogenital Complications

Damage to the urinary tract during proctocolectomy is not very frequent, but it can occur. Ureteral fistulas can develop. Postoperative urinary complications are more often due to damage to the pelvic autonomic nerve plexus or to postoperative pelvic discomfort inhibiting bladder emptying. A neurogenic bladder postoperatively is treated by urethral catheterization initially, followed after a few days by clamping of the catheter to enable bladder function to become reestablished. Urecholine can be used to assist in this. Urinary tract infections should be sought and treated with antibiotics. The perineal wound and the pelvic area should be examined carefully for signs of pelvic abscess formation if urinary difficulties persist for more than about a week postoperatively.

Five to ten percent of men experience impotence or failure of ejaculation after the surgery. Careful dissection of the rectum diminishes the incidence of this complication. In a certain number of patients, the troubles are temporary—in some cases they are probably psychological—but the patient should be made aware of the risks, before surgery. Elderly men are more likely to have postoperative sexual dysfunction than younger men. Women do not suffer as frequently from postoperative sexual dysfunction; in women, pelvic pain resulting from the surgery or from perineal wound infection appears to be more troublesome than neurological damage to the sensation of orgasm. In both sexes, psychological reactions to the presence of the ileostomy can inhibit libido; psychotherapy can often be valuable, with the internist and the surgeon providing additional supportive encouragement. Preoperative psychological preparation for the ileostomy with help to prevent the dual shocks of postoperative pelvic discomfort and sudden mutilation of the body.

Cardiopulmonary Complications

Any major abdominal operation can result in cardiac and pulmonary complications. Postoperative chest infections are a problem, especially in smokers and in patients with preexisting cardiopulmonary disease. Patients with any degree of ischemic heart disease are liable to develop myocardial infarction as a complication of the anesthesia. Postanesthetic arrhythmias can be a problem in any patient. Deep venous thrombosis and pulmonary embolism are postoperative complications that are potentially fatal, and patients with ulcerative colitis are especially prone to them.

Cerebral Complications

Cerebral dysfunction has been noted uncommonly frequently in the postoperative period in patients undergoing proctocolectomy for ulcerative colitis. This complication is mostly seen in patients who have been particularly sick immediately before the surgery, and often these patients have been receiving large doses of steroids. They remain in coma for an unduly long period postoperatively; they often have epileptic seizures (95); and their mental capacity immediately after surgery is subnormal.

Most do recover full mental function in the weeks following these episodes, and it is rare for the epileptic fits to continue. A few, however, have permanent brain damage. The reason for this is unclear, but cerebral edema seems the most likely explanation, related to the hypoxia of the operation combined with preoperative electrolyte imbalance consequent on the diarrhea and the use of corticosteroids. It should be recalled that cerebral venous thrombosis and benign intracranial hypertension are both known complications of ulcerative colitis (Chapter 8).

OTHER SURGICAL APPROACHES

Two-Stage Proctocolectomy

Some surgeons prefer not to perform total proctocolectomy as a single operation, especially if the colectomy is being done urgently. They prefer to leave the rectum in place, with a proximal mucous fistula in the left lower quadrant of the abdomen, and to resect the rectum as an elective procedure a few weeks later. This shortens the time of anesthesia for an acutely ill patient and allows a careful, unhurried subsequent excision of the rectum, using the care required to avoid damaging the pudendal nerves.

Of course, if the patient is bleeding actively from the rectum, this two-stage procedure should not be employed. Other approaches to the two-stage procedure involve leaving the proximal end of the rectal stump (tied) in the pelvis or subcutaneously in the left lower quadrant. This is considered to give a greater risk of perforation, peritonitis, and pelvic abscess formation than if a mucous fistula is fashioned. Even with the mucous fistula, the risk of these perforative complications is a little greater than with a primary resection; but the individual surgeon must assess the risks for himself in his own hands.

Ileostomy and Colostomy in Acute Dilatation of the Colon

An unconventional approach is practiced by Turnbull and colleagues at the Cleveland Clinic (96) in cases of acute toxic dilatation of the colon. The dilatation is relieved by performing two temporary stomas, one a transverse colostomy and the other a distal ileostomy. This is not an approach that most other surgeons or physicians recommend because it involves leaving in place an inflamed colon that remains liable to perforate.

Ileorectal Anastomosis

Some surgeons practice the technique of ileorectal anastomosis as an alternative to proctocolectomy for ulcerative colitis (97). It can be done as a one-stage or a two-stage procedure. When it is performed in two stages, the decision to create the anastomosis can be left until the rectomucous fistula is seen to be uninflamed, although this is possibly a false indication of the situation to be expected following restoration of the flow of bowel contents. The advantages of ileorectal anastomosis are plain, because the patient retains a normal anal passage for the stool. However, this is rarely a normally formed stool, the patients generally having three to six loose motions daily. With this operation, there is much less danger of damage to genitourinary function.

The disadvantage of an ileorectal anastomosis is that the colitis remains in the rectal stump, where it can cause rectal bleeding and diarrhea and where it continues to have carcinogenic potential, although the precancerous field is, admittedly, a fraction of what it would have been prior to the operation. Six-monthly or even three-monthly sigmoidoscopic examinations are essential for the detection of cancer or of epithelial dysplasia (as a precancerous lesion) in the rectal stump. The worst aspect of ileorectal anastomosis is that even in the best hands the increased risk of death as a result of the surgery is roughly three times that of proctocolectomy (mainly due to leakage of bowel contents at the line of anastomosis). And one must bear in mind that one-third or more of patients who are treated with an ileorectal anastomosis will later need a proctectomy with an ileostomy.

One can probably justify an ileocrectal anastomosis in a patient with ulcerative colitis who is otherwise healthy, who has relative sparing of the rectum, and who is between the ages of 30 and 45—older than 30 because the number of years he will have to live with the cancer risk will not be as great as with younger patients, and younger than 45 because of the greater operative risks with increasing age. An obstructing benign stricture may be treated by an ileorectal anastomosis.

Diversionary Ileostomy

Diversionary ileostomy involves the creation of a temporary ileostomy, with the distal opening of the divided ileum being fashioned into a mucous fistula so that the colon is isolated from the flow of bowel contents. The procedure should not be termed a double-barreled ileostomy, because the distal stoma should be placed away from the fecal ileostomy, higher on the abdominal wall so that fecal soiling of the distal stoma does not occur. The isolated colon is perfused with topical steroid solutions for a period of time, usually about a year; and then the continuity of the bowel is restored at another operation.

This procedure is still used, with a certain justification, for some patients with Crohn's disease of the colon; but the results of its use in patients with ulcerative colitis have shown that the activity of the colitis is just as bad after the re-joining as it was prior to the temporary diversion, and the operative risks are significant. The authors can recount the successful use of this procedure in a 6-week-old child with ulcerative colitis; in that instance, the greater operative risks were worth taking because of the dreadful social problems for that particular child, had a permanent ileostomy been created. There may be other similar cases in which a trial of a temporary ileostomy is justifiable, but in general it is not to be recommended.

Partial Colectomy with a Permanent Colostomy

Ulcerative colitis has a tendency to spread to involve the entire colon, even if the proximal colon is apparently spared. Once the rectum is to be removed and the patient must live with a fecal stoma, there is no justification for removing less than the whole colon. The salt- and water-retaining effects of the colonic mucosa are taken over in time by the distal ileum in patients with an ileostomy, and the stool from a colostomy is more often malodorous than that from an ileostomy. Leaving behind the proximal colon in a patient with ulcerative colitis leaves the patient liable to recurrence of the colitis in that part of the bowel, with potential for bleeding, perforation, and development of cancer, as well as lesser disabilities from recurrent ulcerative colitis.

The Continent Ileostomy of Kock

A Swedish surgeon, Kock, has designed a form of ileostomy that is usually continent, so that the patient does not have to wear an ileostomy bag (98). An ileal reservoir is emptied several times a day with a catheter. The distal 50 cm or so of the ileum is made into a fecal reservoir, and the opening is formed into an intussuscepted nipple. The stoma does not spout from the skin. In the most experienced hands, good results are obtained, with continence of the ileostomy. In the United States, this operation is being performed at the Mayo Clinic. However, the procedure must still be considered to be in a phase of evaluation. The excellent surgical group in Leeds, England, reports that of 26 patients treated with the Kock ileostomy 1 developed necrosis of the reservoir, 3 developed fecal fistulas, 1 had volvulus of the reservoir, and there were 3 other cases of intestinal obstruction (99). Patients with ulcerative colitis who are otherwise healthy are candidates for this operation, but they must be aware of the risks. Perhaps they should be encouraged to wait another five years or so for the techniques to be improved.

Magnetic Stoma Devices

There has recently been developed a magnetic type of colostomy appliance, and this may prove applicable to ileostomies also. A magnetic cobalt ring is placed subcutaneously around the stoma, and the patient wears a cobalt plate that remains attached magnetically to the abdominal wall, occluding the stoma. This plate is removed a few times a day to allow emptying of the ileal contents (100).

Rectal Mucosal Stripping

Rectal muscosal stripping is a technique that has been developed by Hampton (101) in Houston, Texas, and is still very much in an experimental stage. The rectum and sigmoid are not resected when the remainder of the large bowel is removed; but the mucosa of the rectosigmoid is stripped down to the submucosa, and granulation tissue is allowed to form. Hampton claims that the mucosa regenerates. An ileostomy is created, and a few months later the ileum is anastomosed to the sigmoid. Hampton claims success so far with seven patients for an unspecified follow-up period (five years is the longest).

THE SURGERY OF LOCAL COMPLICATIONS

Surgical intervention for local complications of ulcerative colitis is fairly straightforward, but good technique is important. Perirectal abscesses require incision and drainage. Perianal fistulas should be laid open, but operations on fistulas should be delayed for a few weeks to allow specific medical therapy for any active colitis. The surgical treatment of hemorrhoids does not appear to be particularly hazardous in ulcerative colitis (85). When the rectal mucosa is inflamed, local surgical procedures become more hazardous. Sometimes the requirement for surgical treatment of a perirectal complication results in a decision to perform total colectomy, if that decision was already close at hand.

17

ILEOSTOMY CARE

The decision to perform total colectomy and ileostomy in patients with ulcerative colitis must be a combined medical and surgical one. Similarly, the care following surgery must involve a combined approach, not only for the immediate postoperative period but also for the years to come.

The physician who has been caring for the person with ulcerative colitis usually knows much more about his patient as a person than does the surgeon, and that physician should have the opportunity of participating in the patient's care after the disease has been surgically cured. The physician should keep himself informed about the details of the ileostomy and ileostomy care, and about the consequent physiological changes.

PREOPERATIVE PREPARATION

Some preoperative preparation is required before an operation that is to result in an ileostomy, not only technical preparation but also psychological preparation of the patient. The latter should be in agreement with the decision and should be looking forward to a life free of disease. If another person with an ileostomy is available to visit the patient, the visit should take place before surgery, to encourage the patient further. The site of the stoma should be selected most carefully with regard to proper fit of the ileostomy appliance. The site should be free of any surgical scar or area of skin disease and should not be close to the umbilicus, the inguinal crease, or the iliac crest (see Chapter 16 and Figure 16–1). Some surgeons have the patient wear the appliance for a day sometime before surgery to assure the best fit (Figure 17–1). The site for the stoma should be marked indelibly on the patient's skin before surgery.

POSTOPERATIVE CARE

The ileostomy does not function for the first few days after surgery; so the stoma is simply covered by a transparent disposable appliance. The color of the stoma should be observed frequently to make sure that it does not darken, indicating that its blood supply may be inadequate. During this immediate postoperative period, the patient must be supported with intravenous fluids and nutrients, and

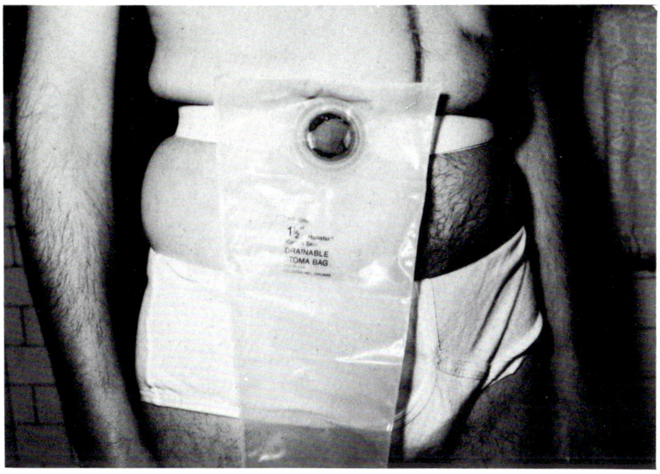

FIGURE 17–1
Patient wearing a disposable ileostomy bag prior to the operation at which an ileostomy is to be created.

he may also need hydrocortisone if he was receiving corticosteroids preoperatively. Details of early postoperative care were discussed in Chapter 16.

Prophylactic skin care is paramount. If the skin was healthy before surgery, it will remain so if not exposed to the corrosive action of the pancreatic enzymes contained in the small bowel fluid. A disposable appliance is placed at the time of surgery and should be replaced immediately if it loosens. At no time should the stoma be covered with dressings.

If the patient has had dermatological disease preoperatively (e.g., eczema or psoriasis), an expert dermatologist must be involved in ileostomy care from the outset. The presence of such a disease is a relative contraindication to performing colectomy with ileostomy in a borderline case and is one instance in which one should seriously consider ileorectal anastomosis, despite its drawbacks (Chapter 16).

EQUIPMENT (Figure 17–2)

Over the past few years, a burgeoning in the number of available appliances and accessories has occurred and will continue to occur, offering the ileostomy patient a wide variety of techniques in caring for and coping with the stoma. Many different manufacturers make excellent appliances. A list can be obtained from a local enterostomal therapist or from the United Ostomy Association in the United States or the Ileostomy Association in Great Britain.

Appliances

Basically, all appliances consist of a pouch with a drainable spout (see Figure 17–2, *center foreground*). That portion of the appliance attached to the skin around

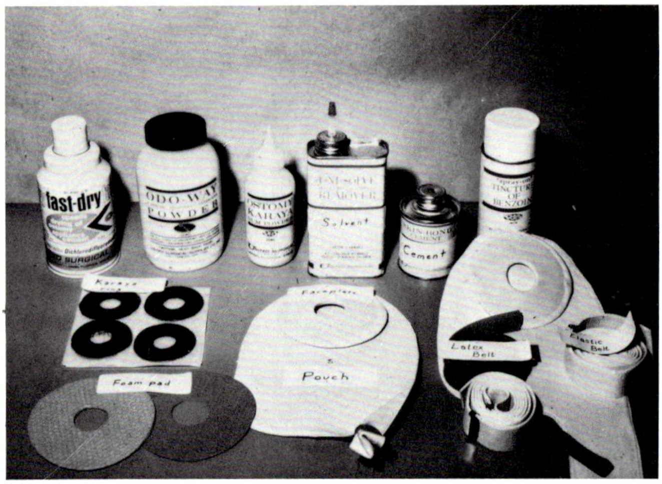

FIGURE 17–2
Typical equipment needed by a patient with an ileostomy who uses a permanent appliance.

the stoma is called the face plate (Figure 17–2, *left center*). Two broad categories of appliances are the *disposable* and the *permanent.* Disposable appliances are used immediately after surgery, as described above, and are made of transparent or opaque plastic (Figure 17–1). The opening of the face plate is supplied with a material to protect the skin, such as a karaya gum washer. A belt helps to hold the bag in place.

Once the postoperative period is over (usually about six weeks), the stoma should have assumed its permanent size and shape. The patient may then elect to obtain a so-called permanent appliance or to continue to use disposables. The chief advantage of the disposables is their convenience. The permanent appliances are less expensive over the long run. Permanent appliances are made of heavy plastic, vinyl, or rubber (Figure 17–2) and can be reused after washing. The face plate may be incorporated into the pouch as a one-piece appliance or may be separate with a removable pouch, making a two-piece appliance. It must be made clear to the patient that "permanent" does not mean that the face plate is never removed—it must be washed every few days. One of the most crucial measures to be taken to avoid stoma problems is the accurate fitting of the appliance to the size of the stoma. Complications arise when the appliance is too large and when it is too small.

Accessories

The mode of attaching the appliance is critical to skin care and hence to the well-being of the ileostomy patient. Leakage of intestinal contents results in excoriation of the peristomal skin. The raw, weeping surface makes application of the face plate extremely difficult. Most face plates are applied to the skin with special, nonallergic cement or with a double-faced adhesive paper disk.

Karaya powder has been used for years to protect the peristomal skin since it is not digested by pancreatic enzymes. Furthermore, the powder will adhere to raw, irritated skin, yielding a dry surface for application of the face plate. Karaya powder is combined with glycerine to make a solid form that can be shaped into rings. The karaya rings have the same protective quality as the powder but are softer and adhere closely to the stoma when placed between the skin and face plate. Newer products such as Stomahesive (E. R. Squibb and Sons, Inc.) and ReliaSeal (Davol Inc.) are synthetic materials that often last longer than karaya rings, though they are more expensive.

The appliance and the protective ring and cement, or the adhesive disk, are the basic needs for the ileostomy patient who changes the entire appliance about once every four or five days. For those patients with special problems, the appliance may need to be changed more frequently. The enterostomal therapist is trained to help the patients with ileostomy problems. Additional equipment that would be helpful in unusual instances includes tincture of benzoin, plastic sprays to prepare the skin, deodorants, and various other products (102).

LOCAL COMPLICATIONS

A properly constructed stoma will give little problem to the patient, whereas a poorly functioning stoma will lead to severe skin irritation and possibly to small bowel obstruction.

Skin Problems

As noted above, prevention of skin irritation by not allowing intestinal contents to touch the peristomal skin is of prime importance. Once irritation has occurred (Figure 17–3), the raw skin must be allowed to heal; yet it must still submit to the

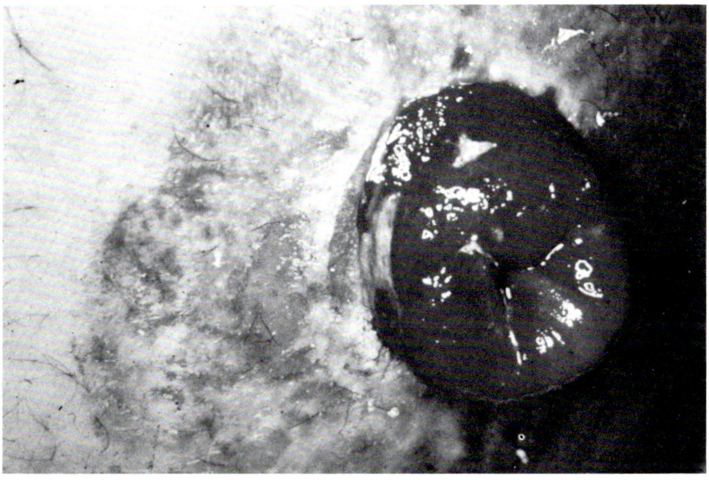

FIGURE 17–3
Dermatitis surrounding an ileostomy.

application of the pouch to prevent further irritation. Within a short time, alteration of the epidermis may occur, further complicating the problem.

Karaya powder or rings, synthetic materials, and even a paste made from antacids have been useful in healing excoriated skin. Patients often return to disposable appliances during the period the skin is irritated, since these appliances have protective materials incorporated in the design and are easy to change frequently. Occasionally, local corticosteroids are helpful in healing certain irritations, while nystatin ointment or powder (Mycostatin) can help heal monilial overgrowth.

There are specific "don'ts" with regard to peristomal skin irritation: 1) *Don't* remove the appliance and apply dressings. This will allow further soilage and damage from intestinal contents. 2) *Don't* apply zinc oxide or aluminum paste. These substances do not protect the skin and prevent proper adherence of the appliance.

Blockage by Food

Frequently the bowel is narrowed as the ileostomy passes through the abdominal wall, creating a potential site for blockage by food. Those foods high in cellulose, such as peanuts, popcorn, coconut, corn-on-the-cob, celery, water chestnuts, and bean sprouts, that are not digested by pancreatic enzymes will exit from the bowel essentially unchanged. If ingested in large amounts, these high-cellulose foods will conglomerate and create a mechanical small bowel obstruction at the point close to the ileostomy where the intestine passes through the abdominal wall. If this opening is large enough, there will be no problem with any type of food, whereas if the opening is too small, recurrent blockage becomes a problem.

Again, prevention is the best therapy. Patients should be cautioned against eating those foods high in cellulose. The stoma can be checked for stenosis by the physician gently inserting his little finger into the stoma. If the finger can be inserted at full length, the lumen is not stenotic. If a narrowing is encountered at the fascial line, the patient is strongly warned about the possibility of intestinal obstruction due to food.

Once a food blockage has occurred, the bowel may be irrigated gently with saline to break up the food aggregate. Surgery is rarely indicated in this situation, although actual small bowel obstruction from other causes, such as adhesions, internal hernias, or volvulus, must be excluded.

Prestomal Intestinal Obstruction

Besides food blockage, which can nearly always be corrected without surgery, patients with ileostomy are also liable to develop intestinal obstruction due to intra-abdominal mechanical complications—adhesions or herniation of the ileum into the lateral space (see Chapter 16). Intermittent obstruction may manifest itself by ileostomy diarrhea, caused by the sudden rush of temporarily backed up fluid.

Stomal Abnormalities

The ileostomy is created by pulling several centimeters of ileum through an opening in the abdominal wall and folding the end of the bowel over itself to create a mucosa-covered stoma (93). The ileostomy should protrude about 2 cm beyond the abdominal wall, in contrast to the flush colostomy. If a stoma is constructed improperly or undergoes changes due to scarring, certain ileostomy complications arise. The most common problems are retraction and stenosis of the stoma, often occurring together. Prolapse of the stoma is more serious.

Retraction

Retraction refers to the stoma being pulled into the abdominal cavity, probably by scarring; an excessively short stoma is thereby created, so that the intestinal contents cannot be directed into the appliance properly. The ileal effluent then accumulates around the stoma and undermines the seal of the face plate, causing leakage and skin irritation. A stoma may have been created too short in the first place, and this will result in the same problem. The stenotic stoma is described above. Revision of the stoma is required when either of these two problems occurs; they cannot be dealt with merely by manipulating the appliance or changing accessories. The stoma can then be reformed without changing its location.

Prolapse

Prolapse is caused by failure of the serosal surface of the stoma to adhere subcutaneously, together with failure of fixation of the distal ileum within the peritoneum, but with the mucosa-skin interface secure, so that the bowel prolapses like a sleeve being turned inside out. On the occurrence of straining, or even as a spontaneous occurrence, several centimeters of the bowel may come out through the stoma, suddenly pushing off the appliance. If the bowel is allowed to remain prolapsed, it may become edematous and compromise its own blood supply; thus, this condition can lead to gangrene. Therefore, a prolapsed stoma must be replaced immediately. If prolapse occurs too frequently, a surgical revision is required and the stoma must be moved to another site since the opening in the abdominal wall is usually too large.

ILEOSTOMY FLUID LOSS

The main physiological impact of the loss of the colon is a decreased ability to reabsorb water and sodium. Potassium loss is usually not a significant problem. The ileostomy patient is often mildly salt-depleted and dehydrated, for which he should compensate by making a deliberate effort to drink more water and adding extra salt. Normally, the ileostomy patient empties the appliance four to six times daily; the average ileostomy output is 1 liter of fluid. If a significant amount of distal ileum has been removed, the fluid loss is greater. An increase in ileostomy output is often accompanied by a concomitant decrease in urine flow due to depletion of the intravascular volume. The patient should be taught to observe and report an increased ileal flow and also any noticeable diminution in urinary volume.

Ileostomy Diarrhea

The ileostomy effluent should decline in volume in the weeks following surgery (due to ileal adaptation taking over the reabsorptive role of the colon) and should then solidify. Persistence or recurrence of a fluid effluent may be an indication of 1) an acute or subacute infectious gastroenteritis in the small bowel; 2) intermittent or partial small intestinal obstruction; 3) recurrence of Crohn's disease in a patient misdiagnosed as having ulcerative colitis; 4) mild prestomal ileitis (Chapter 16)—but this does not cause an increased volume of fluid even if it is liquid and slightly bloody; 5) a completely unrelated diarrhea (e.g., caused by hypolactasia or chronic pancreatitis), which may manifest itself as a result of the colectomy; or 6) a factor due to none of these—"nonspecific."

A plain abdominal X-ray should be taken to exclude intestinal obstruction; and if the ileostomy diarrhea persists for more than one to two weeks, a small bowel follow-through barium X-ray study should be performed to exclude Crohn's disease or another small intestinal disease. Culture and microscopy of the ileostomy fluid are rarely helpful in diagnosing infectious gastroenteritis—only *Shigella, Salmonella,* and *Giardia lamblia* infections can be diagnosed by routine examination of this fluid.

Gastroenteritis

The absence of the colon still leaves the ileostomy patient vulnerable to infectious gastroenteritis. The vomiting and the ileostomy diarrhea that accompany such infection often have a severe impact and result in a much more severe dehydration than in the normal adult. If fluids can be taken orally, a physiological saline can be made up by adding a teaspoon each of salt and baking soda to a quart of water, with a twist of lemon for flavor. The patient should ingest about the same quantity as the estimated loss from the stoma. If signs of hypovolemia are present, a brief course of intravenous fluids with salt and water is indicated, even for an outpatient in an emergency room.

Severe or Persistent Ileostomy Diarrhea

Patients with severe ileostomy diarrhea may have to be admitted to the hospital for intravenous fluid therapy. Fluid balance charts must be kept carefully, and it may be necessary to send a sample of the ileostomy fluid to the laboratory for estimation of its sodium and potassium concentrations.

For persistent ileostomy diarrhea, often of the "nonspecific" type, it is worth while prescribing medications to slow down the motor function of the small intestine. Lomotil, codeine, and loperamide (Imodium) have all been shown to be effective, although a particular patient may do best with one of these rather than another in the group. If the diarrhea does not respond to medication, the patient should certainly have a further gastrointestinal investigation.

SYSTEMIC COMPLICATIONS

Kidney Stones

The person with an ileostomy is 20 times more prone to kidney stones than the normal adult. The state of mild chronic dehydration creates a concentrated urine, allowing the precipitation of phosphate, oxalate, and uric acid stones (see Chapter 8).

Obesity

Since the colon does not participate in food absorption, the patient with an ileostomy will not lose weight unless a significant portion of the terminal ileum has also been removed. In the patient with ulcerative colitis, the terminal ileum is healthy or only superficially diseased. Patients who have been chronically ill or on a special diet for many years and patients who have lost weight following surgery often find great joy in eating and may overshoot the return of weight. Unhappily, excess weight is a major problem with many ileostomy patients. One of the unforeseen consequences of obesity is a change in the contour of the abdomen, which may create a problem with fitting the ileostomy appliance. There is no special mode of therapy, and these overweight patients must diet in the same way as persons with a colon. On the other hand, they must be warned that a *sudden* loss of weight associated with ileostomy diarrhea is not a sign of success in their weight-reducing program but may indicate a dangerous situation that may lead to dehydration (see above).

GENERAL HEALTH OF ILEOSTOMY PATIENTS

In the first year following the creation of the ileostomy, there is a very small mortality due to surgical complications, mainly intestinal obstruction. After that first year, the overall life expectancy is excellent (although patients in whom carcinoma was present in the colon must be exculded from this statement) (103). The only disease that seems more common than in the general community is the development of renal calculi. Gallstones do not appear to be particularly common in patients having an ileostomy for ulcerative colitis. The patients still remain liable to illness and mortality from those extracolonic complications of ulcerative colitis—ankylosing spondylitis and the hepatobiliary disorders (Chapter 8)—which do not regularly remit following colectomy.

SOCIAL AND PSYCHOLOGICAL PROBLEMS

The great majority of patients with an ileostomy manage to continue leading normal lives. They can engage in almost every employment and social activity except for certain sports. Most sports are possible, including swimming, but body-contact sports such as American football and rugby must be forbidden. Since ileostomy diarrhea can be sudden in its onset and dangerously dehydrating, patients should not be far from medical help. They should not trek up the Amazon! Ileostomy patients have included ballerinas and surgeons. At least one famous film star has an ileostomy.

The modern appliances fit closely to the skin, and if the most clinging and see-through fashions are avoided, the patient should be able to lead his or her life without the existence of the ileostomy being discernable at work or in social gatherings. Odors are rarely a problem with ileostomies, but when an odor is detectable, there are deodorants available that can be placed in the stoma bag. The presence of an odor should be an indication to check the tightness of the fit of the appliance.

Naturally, this stance of normality cannot be carried into the patient's sexual relationships. These are a problem, but a remarkable number of spouses come to terms with the situation. Many recall the days of the patient's ill health from ulcerative colitis and are relieved by the solution of that aspect. Ileostomy associations and marriage counselors can play important roles in helping with the sexual problems of ileostomy patients.

Suicide is a risk in patients with an ileostomy, though not a great risk: there were only two suicides in Ritchie's series of over 300 patients (103). In fact, suicide is also a risk in symptomatic ulcerative colitis (104).

18

ULCERATIVE COLITIS IN CHILDHOOD

Although ulcerative colitis is commoner in adults and commonest in the late teens and in the 20s, it is certainly a disease that can occur in children of any age, although it is less frequent in the youngest age group. The authors have experience of a well-documented case in a baby 6 weeks old, and other cases have been reported in children under 1 year. Gastroenteritis is such a prevalent condition among babies that ulcerative colitis may not be considered as a possible diagnosis. The occurrence of bloody diarrhea in a child should be an indication for a sigmoidoscopic examination (and a biopsy may be justified). Ulcerative colitis may then be apparent.

The disease has a tendency to be more severe in children than in adults. Total colonic involvement with ulcerative colitis is commoner in children than among adults (more than 50% in Truelove's series), and the onset of the disease in childhood is itself an increased risk factor for the development of colonic carcinoma, additional to the risk factors of extensive anatomical involvement and of long duration of the disease (the latter inevitable if the colitis starts in childhood) (35).

The symptoms, signs, and management of ulcerative colitis in children are in general no different from those in adults, although some of the details have to be considered a little differently in children.

CONSIDERATIONS RELATED TO THE CHILD'S PERSONALITY

An infant cannot communicate the localization of abdominal pain, although a parent or a pediatrician can often suspect this. Diarrhea with or without bleeding is the usual presentation of ulcerative colitis, and the examination of an infant's stools is a normal event. In the 3 to 10 age group, there is generally little difficulty in the parents' discovering a bowel disturbance. The older child and adolescent, on the other hand, are learning privacy and independence and may not report rectal bleeding or diarrhea, out of fear of the social consequences of being abnormal, out of fear of the discomforts of the inevitable medical investigations and treatments, or simply out of embarrassment that is common among adolescents.

Investigations

Sigmoidoscopies, barium enema X-ray examinations, and colonoscopies pose problems when the patient is a child. Pediatric instruments are available and should be used. Special tact is needed when performing these studies on children. Occasionally, general anesthesia needs to be employed in order to undertake sigmoidoscopy or colonoscopy. Many children are remarkably brave, more so than some young adults. Although for children the physician needs to be a little more sparing in the use of follow-up studies than would be the case for adults, the tendency, the authors find, is to be excessively sparing to the detriment of the correct management of those children who have a serious but treatable disorder. Sigmoidoscopy and barium enema X-ray study should never be omitted in the evaluation of disease in a child with ulcerative colitis, unless the child is being seen on referral and the studies have already been done by a reputable specialist. The consequences to the child of a diagnosis of ulcerative colitis are such that histological confirmation with a biopsy is essential. The existence of a biopsy slide may spare the child a future sigmoidoscopy when a new specialist is consulted.

Psychological Factors

The role of psychological factors in the etiology of ulcerative colitis has been discussed in Chapter 3. One frequently gets a feeling that children with ulcerative colitis have overprotective parents, but often this is a natural reaction by the parents to a child with this disease and its symptoms. The parent-child relationships do need special handling when ulcerative colitis occurs in children and in teenagers. It is important for the physician to try to convince the parents that there should be no guilt feeling on their part. The doubts expressed in the medical literature about the bearing of psychological factors on ulcerative colitis can be relayed to the parents to dispel the lay impression that ulcerative colitis is a "psychosomatic" disorder.

It often helps to see the child and the parents separately, as well as together. Seeing the child alone can be very revealing with regard to the actual nature of the symptoms, as well as in the matter of relationships and stresses at home, school, and elsewhere. It also allows the physician to build a rapport with the child directly and without inevitable parental interference. The authors have been struck with how often the parents resent the physician's seeing the child alone. Such a situation requires careful handling, and the parents must be reassured at the outset that they too will be consulted and informed fully.

CONSIDERATIONS RELATED TO THE CHILD'S SIZE

The same drugs are used in children as in adults, although doses are normally proportionately less. As a rule of thumb, one can say that children under 2 receive one-quarter of the adult dose of steroids and sulfasalazine; that children from 2 to 8 are given one-half the adult dose; and that children from 8 to 12 receive three-quarters of the dose, over 12s being treated as adults.

Alternate-day steroids are used more often by pediatricians than by physicians treating adults, and the authors recommend this when the disease is not severe and an attack is on the wane. The use of alternate-day steroids has been discussed in Chapter 13. The authors are not particularly in favor of using steroids in children, even on alternate days, for more than about three months.

CONSIDERATIONS RELATED TO PREPUBERTY

Growth retardation is not uncommon among children with ulcerative colitis, but fortunately it is by no means as frequent as among children with Crohn's disease. Growth should be assessed by the child's height, rather than the weight; and the height should be compared with that predicted, taking into account the heights of the parents.

Malabsorption is not a feature of ulcerative colitis because the small intestine is not involved in this disease. Growth retardation in ulcerative colitis is a result of the loss of protein, blood, and possibly other factors from the inflamed colon. Treatment of the colitis itself can be expected to assist in the restoration of normal growth and development. This may not be so simple, because 1) corticosteroids adversely affect growth and pubertal development and 2) the child may be so malnourished that the normal healing processes of the recovery stage may be impaired.

As far as steroids are concerned, they should be used in the full appropriate doses to inhibit the inflammatory colitis, but in courses of no more than three months or so. Long-term steroid medication is particularly undesirable in children because of the effects of steroids on growth. Even in adults, many physicians consider that proctocolectomy should be performed rather than maintaining a patient on steroids, and in the case of children this view is even more certain.

Azathioprine can be used as a "steroid-sparing" drug. The potential side effects of long-term azathioprine therapy (oncogenesis and genetic damage) should be considered, but they are not great. In children, the medium-term use of azathioprine (six months to two years) is probably preferable to a larger dose of steroids, and it may avoid the need for a colectomy.

British physicians now have the opportunity to try children on disodium cromoglycate (Nalcrom) (see Chapter 13).

Malnutrition can be corrected by a high-calorie, high-protein oral diet or by intravenous hyperalimentation, but there is not a great chance of the success of hyperalimentation in a child with more than moderately active ulcerative colitis. The malnourished child whose disease is brought into a relative remission, whether or not colectomy is to follow, can be restored to better health and better ability to withstand the risks of the colectomy operation by a period of parenteral hyperalimentation; but there are not many such cases.

Following proctocolectomy, the child who has suffered from growth impairment generally catches up rapidly with his or her expected growth curve, *provided that the child was not allowed to pass through puberty while stunted.* Postpubertal growth-stunted teenagers do have a growth spurt, but they often do not attain their expected height. The discontinuance of steroids and the consideration of a colectomy become more urgent the closer a child is to puberty.

COLECTOMY IN CHILDREN

The operation of choice for children with ulcerative colitis who have not responded to medical management is proctocolectomy with a permanent ileostomy. Ileorectal anastomosis should not be attempted in children because of its inherent dangers, its ineffectiveness in many cases, and particularly its long-term disadvantages (see Chapter 16). A temporary diversionary ileostomy is sometimes justifiable in children (Chapter 16).

Ileostomy

The parents are generally more fearful about an ileostomy than the child is. Children are relatively adaptable, and they learn quickly how to deal with the ileostomy appliances. Once the child and its parents realize how well the child has become after surgery, there is generally not a great deal of difficulty in accepting the ileostomy. Pediatric-size appliances are available. Ileostomy associations are very supportive of children with ileostomies and of their parents, and the young often become active members. Children nowadays can be encouraged in the hope that continent ileostomies may be perfected soon enough to be applicable to them.

The need for an ileostomy in a child is often denied by the parents, even to the extent of the parents' denying the existence of rectal bleeding when it is present. The parents should be encouraged to take the child to well-known medical centers and for reputable second opinions, though not if the activity of the colitis is considered dangerous or if time is going to be lost at the expense of growth and development. Other young people with ileostomies should meet with the child, and their respective parents can meet with each other.

The surgical technique is similar to that in an adult, although, of course, on a smaller scale. An experienced colonic surgeon who mainly deals with adult cases is probably preferable to a pediatric surgeon without a wide experience of colonic surgery.

THE OUTCOME OF ULCERATIVE COLITIS IN CHILDREN

Although ulcerative colitis is more often severe than mild in childhood, some encouraging results have been reported from the diligent management of such children. Truelove has reported his experience with 57 children under the age of 16 who had ulcerative colitis more extensive than just a proctitis, with a mean follow-up of over six years (105). There was only 1 death; 10 others had an ileostomy (temporary in 2 cases); 1 patient had a portacaval shunt for portal hypertension; and 45 were living relatively normal lives without an ileostomy. Other physicians have not reported quite such good results. It may be that a child with ulcerative colitis should be treated by a gastroenterologist experienced in that disease rather than by a general pediatrician with less experience of inflammatory bowel disease.

19

ULCERATIVE COLITIS AND PREGNANCY

The role of pregnancy as a factor that can aggravate ulcerative colitis has already been mentioned in Chapter 13. In fact, a pregnancy can aggravate or improve ulcerative colitis, almost certainly because of the changes in circulating steroidal hormones that take place in pregnancy. It was the improvement noted in pregnant women suffering from bronchial asthma that led to the use of adrenal corticosteroids in that disease and then in other diseases in which allergy was believed to play a role, including ulcerative colitis.

THE NATURAL HISTORY OF ULCERATIVE COLITIS DURING PREGNANCY

Ulcerative Colitis Prior to Pregnancy

Colitis in Remission

In the published series, approximately one-third of women with ulcerative colitis whose disease is in remission when they become pregnant will have a relapse of the disease during the pregnancy or in the puerperium. However, De Dombal and co-workers (106) have made the important point that a relapse rate of that order in a 10- to 12-month period is usual among women with ulcerative colitis in their 20s and early 30s. In other words, a woman with ulcerative colitis has really no greater chance of a relapse by becoming pregnant, if her disease is in remission at the beginning of the pregnancy. This refers to the total relapse rate in the pregnancy-puerperium period. The situation does vary from trimester to trimester. The relapse rate is greater than normal in the first trimester and even more so in the puerperium, whereas it is lower than normal in the second and third trimesters. Also, the severity of ulcerative colitis relapsing in the first trimester and in the puerperium tends to be greater than usual (particularly if the relapse occurs in the puerperium). This means that the total disease activity of ulcerative colitis during a 12-month period that includes a pregnancy is apt to be worse than in a similar period when there is no pregnancy.

Active Colitis

If the ulcerative colitis is active at the beginning of pregnancy, even if only mildly, there is deterioration in the colitis in two-thirds of patients as a result of the pregnancy. This deterioration is usually in the first trimester, whereas the colitis frequently improves in the second and third trimesters, becoming more severe again in the postpartum period in patients whose colitis has remained active, and sometimes recrudescing in those in whom it has remitted in the latter trimesters. In the one-third of patients whose ulcerative colitis does not deteriorate, a remission can be quite a striking consequence of the pregnancy.

First Attack During Pregnancy or the Puerperium

Pregnancy or the puerperium is frequently a period in which women have their first attack of ulcerative colitis. Again, the colitis is most likely to occur and to be more severe in the first trimester, and less likely to occur and to be more severe in the second and third trimesters; and then there is another peak for onset and severity immediately postpartum. During the pregnancy, the course of the colitis tends to be more severe than usual; and ulcerative colitis commencing in the postpartum period has a tendency to be particularly severe.

EFFECT OF THE COLITIS ON THE FETUS

Observations on the outcome of pregnancy in patients with active ulcerative colitis, in whom colectomy was avoided, have not shown any marked increase in fetal loss above expected levels, either through spontaneous abortion or through stillbirth (106, 107). Fetal death is known to result in individual women with severe cases of ulcerative colitis, especially when colectomy becomes necessary.

EFFECTS ON THE FETUS OF DRUGS USED IN ULCERATIVE COLITIS

One is rightly cautious about using any medication for ulcerative colitis in a woman who is or who may be pregnant. From what is known about the cellular actions of corticosteroids, sulfasalazine, and azathioprine, one might expect these three drugs to be potentially harmful to the fetus. However, there have been no reports clearly implicating any of them as teratogenic agents or as influencing pregnancy adversely in any other way. Nevertheless, one must be confident that specific drugs are indicated during pregnancy when the course of the ulcerative colitis is such as to require them.

Azathioprine is an immunosuppressant known to cause bone marrow suppression, and there are well-documented instances of tumor induction when it was used in renal transplant patients. It is a drug which, on theoretical grounds at least, should be avoided in pregnancy. It can even be said that it has been wisely avoided in pregnancy, so much that there has been insufficient experience of its use in pregnancy and one cannot be comfortable about the lack of reported toxicity. On the other hand, considerable numbers of women must have become pregnant while they were taking the drug, and no reports of teratogenicity are available. The authors do not routinely recommend therapeutic abortion in patients who become pregnant while taking azathioprine, but they would be sympathetic to a patient's desire for an abortion if she were anxious about possible harm to the fetus.

Corticosteroids have been shown to be teratogenic in rats and also in monkeys. Large doses were used in these experiments (108); and cleft palate has been reported in the babies of a small number of women who were treated during pregnancy with large doses of steroids (109). Once again, the authors' conclusion is that steroids are relatively safe but that the physician must be confident that they are really indicated in the dose in which they are to be used before he prescribes them for a pregnant woman. The patient's anxieties should not be aggravated, but the pregnant patient should be told not to alter her steroid dosage (or the dosage of any medication) without reference to her physician.

Sulfasalazine has been used for several decades in pregnant women, and no harmful effects have been reported; however, there remains the possibility that the sulfonamide component may lead to kernicterus in the neonate.

Cromolyn is absorbed to a very small extent and will probably prove to be safe in pregnancy. However, there are insufficient data to permit its use in pregnancy at present.

It should be remembered that oral iron preparations, which are prescribed routinely by many obstetricians, can cause exacerbation of ulcerative colitis; and therefore iron should not be given to pregnant women with a history of ulcerative colitis unless they become significantly anemic due to iron deficiency. If the patient is anemic, the dangers of the anemia outweigh the risks of giving iron. However, if a patient with active colitis gives a history of previous exacerbation of her ulcerative colitis by oral iron preparations, it is probably better to use intravenous or intramuscular iron rather than oral iron.

INVESTIGATION OF THE BOWEL IN A PREGNANT PATIENT

X-rays

Examinations that involve X-radiation in a pregnant woman carry risks of fetal damage. These risks are greater in the first 8 to 12 weeks of pregnancy than in later trimesters. In a woman with a firm diagnosis of ulcerative colitis who is possibly or certainly pregnant, colon X-ray studies should not be performed unless a critical decision (e.g., a colectomy) is dependent upon information that can only be derived from such a study. Barium enema X-rays show the extent of colitis, but the physician can usually draw sufficient information from the ill patient's clinical state and the appearance of her rectum on sigmoidoscopy. If toxic dilatation of the colon is suspected, it is justifiable to take a plain abdominal X-ray, but it is unusual for an experienced physician to need to have barium enema X-ray films taken of a pregnant woman.

Sigmoidoscopy

Sigmoidoscopy can generally be performed safely during pregnancy provided that the instrument is inserted gently and no deeper than is absolutely necessary to assess the severity of inflammation of the rectal mucosa. It should not normally be necessary to insert the instrument beyond 10 to 15 cm in a pregnant woman, unless limited rectosigmoid involvement rather than more extensive colitis is the clinical impression. Examination of the sigmoid can be achieved with less disturbance to the pelvis by the use of a flexible fiberoptic colonoscope or sigmoidoscope to perform a limited examination of the sigmoid.

Fiberoptic Colonoscopy

Fiberoptic colonoscopy in pregnancy should in general be confined to examination of the rectosigmoid region. Fluoroscopy should, of course, be avoided. The colonoscopic examination should be terminated if the instrument does not advance easily and painlessly. There should not be many instances when such an examination is required during pregnancy.

TREATMENT OF ULCERATIVE COLITIS DURING PREGNANCY

Because of the points discussed above, some physicians are hesitant to use specific medications to treat ulcerative colitis occurring during pregnancy. The authors take the opposite view, that a pregnant patient with a well-documented history of active ulcerative colitis, however mild, is at greater risk from the consequences of inadequately treated colitis than from the use of steroids or sulfasalazine. The authors prescribe medical treatment for these patients in the same way as if they were not pregnant (except that the use of azathioprine is avoided). The authors are particularly diligent about following patients with ulcerative colitis when they become pregnant; and every flare-up of the disease is treated, with no waiting for a possible natural remission, as one might do if the patient were not pregnant.

Surgery During Pregnancy

Naturally, one would consider colectomy in a pregnant patient only if it were really necessary. Semielective surgery for patients with chronic troublesome disease is inappropriate during pregnancy. However, colectomy may become necessary during pregnancy when a severe flare-up is uncontrolled by medical management. The surgery is very hazardous for the fetus, with spontaneous abortion being very common afterwards; but there should be no additional risk to the mother as a result of being pregnant. Because of the risk to the fetus, the authors are that much more persistent with medical therapy than they might otherwise be, although not to the extent of putting the mother's life at significant additional risk. The extent to which the child is wanted can become a factor to consider in some cases: one might be less persistent with medical therapy to avoid surgery if the child were not really wanted by the parents. However, the situation is not quite so straightforward, because of the likelihood of a remission of the colitis following the pregnancy and postpartum period; so attempts to avoid surgery should be greater than usual, even if the survival of the baby is not considered important.

Some surgeons have recommended lesser procedures than total proctocolectomy for pregnant patients with ulcerative colitis. A subtotal colectomy, leaving behind a rectomucous fistula, is an appropriate operation in a pregnant woman, avoiding surgery in the pelvis. It should only be done, however, if the rectum is seen to be only mildly inflamed on sigmoidoscopy. The creation of a temporary relieving ileostomy without any form of colectomy is not recommended, because the severely inflamed colon still presents risks to the patient.

THERAPEUTIC ABORTION

Although the pregnancy may be the cause of an exacerbation or of a first attack of ulcerative colitis, generally it is of little help to terminate the pregnancy in order to bring the colitis under control. Studies have shown that in two-thirds of such cases there was no improvement in the colitis following the termination of the pregnancy (106). On the other hand, one-third of patients do improve, so that therapeutic abortion can be justified if the parents are not concerned about the continuance of the pregnancy.

PREGNANCY FOLLOWING COLECTOMY

Pregnancy Following Subtotal Colectomy

It is unusual to encounter a pregnant woman who has had a subtotal colectomy, because few young women with ulcerative colitis are treated with this procedure. The creation of the ileorectal anastomosis in the pelvic region can cause obstetrical difficulties and often results in a cesarean section being required. With continued presence of the rectum in these patients, there is a site where the colitis can recur during pregnancy or in the postpartum period; and there is considerable likelihood of such a recurrence. For these reasons, the possibility of future pregnancy should probably contraindicate ileorectal anastomosis, even if it were feasible by other criteria.

Pregnancy with an Ileostomy

It is more common to encounter a pregnant woman with an ileostomy, and the condition presents a number of difficulties. The one that the male physician tends to forget is the problem of dealing with the ileostomy stoma in the presence of the protuberant abdomen of pregnancy. In the late stages of pregnancy, the woman often needs a mirror in order to see the stoma and to dress it and change the bag.

Structural problems often affect the stoma during pregnancy. The fetus displaces the stoma, and the increased intra-abdominal pressure can cause ileal prolapse. Local surgery may be needed to deal with this. Intestinal obstruction is more common in an ileostomy patient who is pregnant than in an ileostomy patient who is not pregnant. The presence of the fetus increases the likelihood of trouble from postoperative adhesions, of volvulus, and of herniation of the bowel into the lateral space of the peritoneum.

There can also be difficulties at delivery. One-half of such women do achieve vaginal delivery. Obstetric forceps are usually required, and a good-sized episiotomy should be performed. The remainder of these women require cesarean section (110).

Patients with an ileostomy need not be told they must avoid becoming pregnant. Those who already have two or three children should be informed of the additional risks of pregnancy with an ileostomy; but the outcome of such pregnancies is, overall, fairly good. The first year following a proctocolectomy is the most dangerous from the point of view of the development of ileostomy complications, and so the authors normally tell patients with an ileostomy to avoid becoming pregnant for the first 12 months. After that, they should be assured that with good management there is a high chance of a successful pregnancy.

AVOIDANCE OF PREGNANCY

Contraception

From the above discussion, the conclusion is that a pregnancy does increase somewhat the risks inherent in suffering from ulcerative colitis and should therefore be avoided if there is no strong desire to have a child. For women with ulcerative colitis who do wish to have children, it is desirable that there elapse a period of the order of six months without significant disease activity before pregnancy is embarked upon. Following a proctocolectomy with an ileostomy, a period of 12 months should elapse before the patient should consider becoming pregnant. This implies that contraception should be as effective as possible in patients who have had ulcerative colitis who do not wish to become pregnant.

The methods available for contraception should be well known, but there is a surprising ignorance about them in the general community. The physician taking care of a woman with ulcerative colitis should bring up the question of contraception and the desire for children, and he should be sure that the patient receives good professional advice on the means of contraception. The most effective means is the contraceptive pill; but this has risks in patients who have had ulcerative colitis, risks of causing a flare-up of the colitis, and risks of thromboembolism in a patient whose colitis itself predisposes to thromboembolism. These risks are not great and are small compared with the risks of pregnancy in a woman with ulcerative colitis. The authors' view is that if other means of contraception are unacceptable to the patient or if it is considered that they may be less effective (taking into account the severity of the patient's colitis), the balance of risks usually turns out in favor of oral contraceptives. The intrauterine contraceptive device (IUCD) carries small risks of pelvic infection in any woman who uses it and is probably, therefore, not a good method to choose for a woman who has inflammatory bowel disease. Mechanical barrier methods are harmless, but they are often unacceptable; furthermore, they are not always reliable in preventing pregnancy. Contraceptive jellies and creams are probably the least effective means of contraception. Thus, the choice of a method of contraception has to be a compromise between the risks and the feelings of the patient and her husband.

Termination of Pregnancy

Whatever the moral considerations, there is no doubt that therapeutic termination of pregnancy is the manner in which many women today avoid having children. No data are available implying that women with inactive ulcerative colitis are at increased risk of a recrudescence of the disease as a result of a therapeutic abortion. It is difficult to say whether or not it is any more advisable for a woman with a history of ulcerative colitis to undergo an abortion for a child that is not strongly desired than it is for an otherwise healthy woman. The authors have had as patients young women with ulcerative colitis that has been difficult to control, who have then become pregnant either out of wedlock or in some other situation in which they did not have a strong reason for proceeding through the pregnancy. For such patients, therapeutic abortion has been advised, and such advice can be justified from the general experience of a likely deterioration of the colitis as a result of continuance of the pregnancy.

V

The Natural History

20

PROGNOSIS

The prognosis for a patient with ulcerative colitis can range from excellent to poor, depending upon many factors, which will be discussed. On the average, life expectancy for patients with ulcerative colitis is only about 5 to 10% short of that for the general population; however, around one-fifth of patients will at some time require a colectomy, which usually leaves them with a permanent ileostomy.

It is always important for the physician to be aware of the likely outcome of a disease in his patient and of the effects on the outcome of different forms of therapy. The decision to advise colectomy for ulcerative colitis is not an emergency decision in about one-half of cases; therefore, the assessment of the prognosis with and without surgery is an important exercise prior to recommendation of such an operation.

The patient with ulcerative colitis and his family normally want to know the meaning of the disease in terms of future expectations. In most instances, the best course is to advise the patient fully of the likely prognosis. This is important in two particular situations. First, a patient with mild disease may be unduly fearful for the future because of what he reads and hears about ulcerative colitis, especially with regard to a permanent ileostomy. He can be alarmed by the experiences of other patients he meets in outpatient clinics and in hospital wards. If he does indeed have mild colitis, he needs vigorous reassurance of the benign nature of that form of the disease; and it may be appropriate to inform him of the outcome of more severe disease in case he later encounters patients with worse colitis and feels that his physician has not told him fully of the prognosis. The opposite situation is the patient with severe disease who clearly would benefit from a colectomy, who is resisting having the operation on account of an underappreciation of the severity and danger of his situation and of the improved prognosis following the surgery.

The prognosis in ulcerative colitis does not merely define the mean life expectancy. One needs to know and to recount to the patient something about the graphical shape of the survival curve. The anticipated quality of life is an important dimension of the prognosis. The patient will want to know whether or not he will need a colectomy with an ileostomy, how many hospitalizations he may need, how disabled he will be, and how much bowel discomfort he can expect to endure. He will want to make sensible financial plans.

FACTORS THAT AFFECT PROGNOSIS

The expectancy for survival, for freedom from symptoms and complications, and for freedom from surgery and an ileostomy all run parallel to one another. Following is a discussion of the various factors that indicate a better or a worse outlook.

Severity of the Disease

The more severe the general activity of the disease and the more ill the patient is, the worse is the prognosis.

Intensity of the Inflammation

Severe inflammation of affected areas of the colon, as judged sigmoidoscopically, colonoscopically, or on barium enema X-ray examination, indicates a worse prognosis than does mild inflammation. Totally inactive disease has a particularly good prognosis.

Extent of Involvement

The greater the length of colon involved in the colitis, the worse is the prognosis. This is an important indicator, because proctitis has a very good prognosis, whereas the prognosis in total colitis is much less favorable. Frequently, colonoscopy now shows disease in areas where the barium enema X-ray appearances are normal. It can be assumed that if colonoscopy shows that radiologically normal bowel is involved in disease, the prognosis is not as good as it would be if the colonoscopy showed a normal mucosa; but it must be noted that reports in the literature before 1972 (or thereabouts) base their estimates of prognosis on the *radiological* extent of the colitis.

Presence of Complications

The presence of local and peripheral complications of ulcerative colitis affects the prognosis unfavorably. Colonic complications indicate severe colonic disease. Frank colonic carcinoma has its own particularly gloomy prognosis, which is generally worse than that for colonic carcinoma in noncolitic patients because of difficulties in diagnosis and because of the tendency to intra-epithelial spread of the cancer. Precancerous dysplastic changes in the colonic mucosa indicate such a high likelihood of the development of malignancy that a prophylactic colectomy is required to restore a reasonable prognosis to a patient in whom these changes are seen.

The presence of the peripheral manifestations of ulcerative colitis—joint, eye, and skin symptoms—indicates at least moderate colitic activity, but otherwise the outcome of the colitis is according to the severity of the colonic involvement. An exception is pyoderma gangrenosum, which is an index for a poorer prognosis. The joint and eye manifestations can of themselves be disabling, and also they may lead the patient to a decision for colectomy sooner than might otherwise have been the case.

Mild hepatitis in association with ulcerative colitis probably indicates mild-to-moderate disease, rather than any more benign form; but it seems that less than 5% of such patients develop clinically significant chronic liver disease. Those who do develop chronic active hepatitis, sclerosing cholangitis, or cirrhosis do have a poorer prognosis than patients free from such a degree of liver involvement. The future of patients with the severer forms of liver involvement often is affected more adversely by their liver disease than by their bowel disease. Bile duct carcinoma as a complication of ulcerative colitis has always been reported to be fatal (39).

History of Previous Disease Activity

As far as the future activity of the colitis is concerned, it seems that the prognosis is more dependent on the current state of the colitis than on the history of previous activity. When the patient is experiencing an attack of the disease, the more severe that particular attack, the worse the prognosis. On the other hand, the patient with a mild attack whose attacks over the years have generally been more severe will not be expected to do as well as the patient whose attacks have all been less severe. The report by Watts and colleagues (111), in which the influence of the current status of the disease was stressed, really took as its index the severity of the worst attack in each year of follow-up. As a guideline, the authors of this book would suggest looking back to the course of the disease over the most recent three years and judging the prognosis on that basis, with disease activity prior to this period being considered much less important. This will enable the physician to make a prognosis for patients in remission. One fact that emerged from Dissanayake and Truelove's double-blind trial of sulfasalazine (68) was that the placebo-treated patients whose previous attack had occurred more than three years earlier had the same relapse rate as the placebo-treated patients whose previous attack had occurred between three months and three years earlier. The one aspect of the prognosis that does depend on the total number of years of the presence of the disease is the risk factor for development of carcinoma of the colon, which increases with the length of the history of the disease and, particularly, with the severity of activity in each year of the disease (35).

The severity of the first attack of ulcerative colitis has been found to correlate with the subsequent course of the colitis. The influence of the severity of the first attacks becomes less as the years go by. A first attack, if severe, is more dangerous in the short term than a relapse of equal severity (112). After the first attack, future attacks tend to be a little less severe. This may be because patients who survive a first attack without surgery are a selected group; but it is more likely to be because of a difference in the reaction of the colon to a first attack compared to a relapse. This was apparent in Jewell and Truelove's controlled trial of the immunosuppressant drug azathioprine in ulcerative colitis, the drug being measurably effective in treating relapses but ineffective in treating a first attack (73). The status of the immune response in a relapse may be different from that in a first attack. Alternatively, or additionally, the tissue reactions in the colon following a first attack may provide resistance or otherwise influence the response to later attacks.

Age

The age of the patient is an important indicator of the prognosis. A young age of onset of ulcerative colitis makes the development of carcinoma more likely than a later age of onset (35). This is in addition to the risk associated with the length of the patient's history of the disease, which will become significant earlier in life in a patient whose disease started at a young age than in patients who were older at the time of their first attack. The age of 40 is probably the optimum age to develop ulcerative colitis (if one had the choice!). Leaving aside the cancer risk, the chance that the activity of the disease will be mild is greatest at this age, and the mortality and need for surgery are least. The disease is likely to be a little more troublesome if the onset is in the 20s; and when the onset is in childhood, there is a considerably greater likelihood of its following a more active course. Nevertheless, many children with ulcerative colitis do well with modern treatment and remain in remission for many years (105), even though the chance of this happening is somewhat less than in adults. In elderly patients, the disease becomes more dangerous (although not necessarily so), with more severe relapses and, particularly, a lower resistance of the patient to the disease and its effects, and especially to surgery, should that be required.

Potentially Avoidable Aggravating Factors

The aggravating factors referred to in Chapter 13 are diet, drugs, infections, psychological factors, and pregnancy. Apart from pregnancy, the studies of the prognosis in ulcerative colitis have not paid attention to the influence of these factors. There is a fund of experience that certain drugs (penicillin, oral iron preparations), some infections, and perhaps psychological factors and personal stresses cause relapse of the disease, but one can say no more than that. Patients with hypolactasia who continue to drink milk have been shown to have more severe attacks than other patients with ulcerative colitis, but their attacks do not seem to be more frequent (23).

Factors Not Shown To Affect Prognosis

Sex, race, and social factors have not been shown to influence the prognosis of ulcerative colitis. There have been no comparative studies to show any differences in prognosis between patients in different parts of the world. Because of the effect of modern medical and surgical therapy (see below), one can presume that without this and without hygiene the outcome might not be as good. Hence social and geographical factors probably do play a small part.

Pregnancy

Pregnancy certainly does influence the activity of ulcerative colitis, as was discussed in Chapter 19. Patients in remission when they become pregnant seem no more likely to relapse during the pregnancy and the puerperium, overall, than comparable patients who do not become pregnant (106). As far as the stage of the pregnancy is concerned, they are less likely to relapse in the second and third trimesters and more likely to relapse in the first trimester and particularly in the puerperium. Women whose colitis is active when they become pregnant fare less well than is normal for colitic women of their age. For all patients with colitis who become pregnant, relapses in the puerperium tend to be more severe than usual. There is no evidence that patients who survive pregnancy and the puerperium have a poorer future prognosis if their colitis was particularly active during that time.

INDEXES OF A POOR OUTCOME IN A GIVEN ATTACK

A severe attack of ulcerative colitis can have a 20% chance of being fatal, the chance being greater if it is the patient's first attack of the disease (112); and it is useful in management to be able to predict which severe attacks are more likely to do badly. Toxic dilatation of the colon puts a severe attack in an exceptionally dangerous category of its own; but short of dilatation, it has been shown that there are three important prognostic indicators, which are fever, hypoalbuminemia, and the frequency of stools in the first 24 hours of hospitalization (prognostic in that order), all indicating a likelihood of a poor outlook (i.e., death or a need for major surgery) (113). A continuing fever after 24 hours is also a poor prognostic sign. Indexes of a good prognosis in a severe attack which have been reported are a rise in the serum gamma globulin level and a fall in the alpha$_2$-globulin (114), and a rise to a peak of the glucosamine synthetase activity in serial rectal biopsy specimens (115).

THE INFLUENCE ON PROGNOSIS OF MODERN TREATMENT

Modern treatment, both medical and surgical, appears to be bringing about a real improvement in the prognosis for patients with ulcerative colitis. This fact, which has appeared in several studies (35, 112), is not an expression of a higher rate of diagnosis of more treatable cases but can be seen particularly in the great reductions in the mortality in moderate attacks which have been reported from several medical centers. The mortality in severe attacks has also been improved, though not as much as in moderate attacks.

Medical Treatment

Corticosteroids and sulfasalazine are certainly effective treatments for ulcerative colitis. The steroids are used in severe attacks, and sulfasalazine is probably not as effective in severe as in moderate and mild attacks; hence, it is probably the steroids that have made the greatest inroads among the forms of medical treatment. Modern supportive medical care, which is especially vital in postoperative periods, must also be an important contributor to the improvement in outlook.

The drugs that are used in treating ulcerative colitis (steroids, sulfasalazine, azathioprine) are not totally safe, but the disadvantages reflected in the very few deaths that can be directly ascribed to the use of these drugs have been more than outweighed by their proved benefits, when they are used correctly.

Surgical Treatment: Colectomy with Ileostomy

Operative Mortality

The operation of total colectomy with ileostomy (one-stage or staged with a rectomucous fistula) has a mortality of itself, which is greatly dependent on the severity of the colitis. The most severely affected patients are operated on as emergencies, either because of complications such as perforation or because medical treatment is considered to have failed. The operative and early postoperative mortality of total colectomy performed as an emergency procedure is roughly 15 to 30%, whereas the mortality in elective colectomy for ulcerative colitis is 2% or less (103). The skill and experience of the surgical team appear to have a large influence on the risk of the procedure. Some of the most experienced surgeons at this operation now have mortality of well under 1%; their results show improvement over the years. In one region of England, the operative mortality in over 30 nonteaching hospitals was roughly twice as great for comparably ill patients as in 2 teaching hospitals in that region (103). In the nonteaching hospitals, the mortality was 2% for elective colectomy, compared with a staggering 60% for emergency colectomy. Elderly patients are at particularly high risk.

Effect of Steroid Therapy on Operative Mortality

An increased incidence of specific postoperative complications in patients who have been receiving corticosteroid therapy has been the experience of many surgeons, but no objective increase in mortality has been reported in comparison to patients who have not received steroids. It would be difficult to define comparable groups, because steroids tend to be used in patients with more severe and more chronic disease.

Long-Term Prognosis Following Ileostomy

Between 10 and 20% of patients with ulcerative colitis who have been treated with a permanent ileostomy will need further surgery. In some of these patients, this will be for intestinal obstruction; in the majority, it will be for the various postileostomy problems that have been discussed in Chapter 17.

There has been some dispute recently as to whether or not some of these patients are experiencing recurrence of their inflammatory bowel disease in the small intestine (116, 117). It is usual to ascribe such recurrences to Crohn's disease which was erroneously diagnosed as ulcerative colitis at the time of the colectomy. The authors favor that view because they have not seen patients in whom the diagnosis on the colectomy specimen was unequivocally that of ulcerative colitis who have subsequently had a definite recurrence of inflammatory bowel disease in the small intestine.

The long-term overall prognosis for patients with an ileostomy for ulcerative colitis seems to be excellent after the first postoperative year (103). There is a significant excess mortality over the normal population, and even compared to the rate in patients surviving a comparable attack of ulcerative colitis with medical treatment alone, during the first year; but (111), after that, the life expectancy in some series has been only a fraction less than that of the general population (103, 112).

Comparative Prognosis for Medical and Surgical Treatment

The group of surgeons from Leeds, England, have proposed on the basis of follow-up of medically treated patients and of the mortality of proctocolectomy in their hands that the prognosis for survival for three years or more beyond an attack in patients with colitis involving the entire colon would be better if colectomy were performed prophylactically than if the physician continued to rely on medical management (111). These are a particularly skillful group of surgeons, and the differences they actually showed in their paper (rather than their projections) were small. Even if their hypothesis were true, as it may be, one has to take into account the quality of survival. Most people will take small risks with their lives for many comforts (such as traveling on modern highways), and most would take some risks with medical treatment rather than live with an ileostomy. These same considerations apply with regard to the operations of ileorectal anastomosis and the Kock continent ileostomy (see below). There is one series that shows a considerably poorer prognosis for patients with ulcerative colitis who have required surgery than for those who have not (112), but these are certainly not comparable groups, the more severely ill patients being those who had surgery in the first place.

The Kock Ileostomy

The Kock ileostomy (98) is designed to produce a continent ileostomy, which in the best hands it succeeds in doing in between one-third and two-thirds of cases (when the patient's colectomy was performed for ulcerative colitis). However, there is an alarming incidence of serious postoperative complications in about one-third of cases (99), which can be presumed to lead to a measurable increase in mortality if the operation is performed on a wider scale.

Ileorectal Anastomosis

As discussed in Chapter 16, on most occasions ileorectal anastomosis is not the best operation for a patient with ulcerative colitis. The reported mortality in the series of 300 patients operated on by Aylett in London (97) was 3 to 4% for elective surgery and 17% for emergency surgery. After a mean of approximately five years of follow-up, 5% of patients who were successfully operated on required a permanent ileostomy. In patients with an ileorectal anastomosis, there also seems to be a higher death rate in the years following surgery than in patients who have a primary ileostomy.

CAUSES OF DEATH IN ULCERATIVE COLITIS

It is useful to consider what are the main causes of death in patients with ulcerative colitis. The majority of patients who die directly as a result of their colitis do so from perforation with ensuing peritonitis, from postsurgical complications, or from massive hemorrhage. Carcinoma of the colon accounts for about 20% of colitis-related deaths (a proportion that is probably rising as patients with ulcerative colitis live longer as a result of modern therapy). A few patients die from carcinoma of the biliary tree, and chronic liver disease accounts for about 5% of deaths. Various infections account for a number of deaths in patients receiving forms of medical therapy such as steroids and immunosuppressants; and there have been deaths from infection acquired by patients receiving parenteral hyperalimentation. Sulfasalazine has been responsible for a few deaths, from granulocytopenia and from exfoliative dermatitis. Venous thromboembolism is not an uncommon cause of death in patients with severe ulcerative colitis. In the series of Morowitz and Kirsner (104), there was a 5% incidence of suicide among the causes of death in patients with ulcerative colitis; a significant number of these patients were receiving steroids.

OVERALL PROGNOSIS

The death rate from a single attack of ulcerative colitis should, with modern treatment, be no more than 5 to 10% in a severe attack, 1 to 2% in a moderate attack, and virtually 0% in a mild attack. The annual death rate among patients with ulcerative colitis is about 1% in patients under 60 years of age and 5% in patients over 60 (111). The 20-year survival of young adults in their first attack is now about 95% of their expected survival rate (Figure 20–1) (112), and it is considerably better than this if the first attack is not severe. In children, on the other hand, the survival after 20 years is only about 60% of that expected in most series, although Truelove (105) has had only 1 death in a series of 57 children he has treated personally.

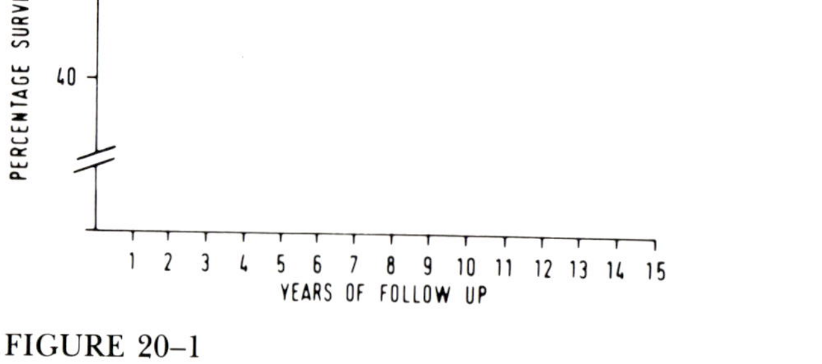

FIGURE 20–1
Survival of patients with ulcerative colitis, excluding those who required surgery in their first attack. Series of Jalan et al (112). (Reproduced by permission of the authors and the Editor of *Gastroenterology*.)

There is a marked tendency for mild colitis to remain mild and for restricted disease to progress little; but in about 10% of patients with mild colitis limited to the rectosigmoid, the disease progresses to total involvement (35). The Cleveland Clinic has reported that 6% of such patients required colectomy in a mean six-year follow-up period (although it should be noted that this reflects the practice of a surgically oriented group) (118). Overall, approximately 20% of patients with ulcerative colitis will require an ileostomy.

The frequency of attacks of ulcerative colitis has been shown to be influenced by treatment with sulfasalazine, which reduces the relapse rate in patients who have intermittent (rather than continuous) disease from about 50% per six months to around 15% per six months (68). It seems that ulcerative colitis always relapses eventually. Edwards and Truelove (35) followed some of their patients for more than 20 years, and all had had at least one relapse by 17 years after their initial attack. In the mid-1960s, Watts and colleagues (111) found that approximately half of their patients were free of symptoms of the disease in any one year.

Most of the studies in the literature on the prognosis of ulcerative colitis are more than 10-years-old and refer to patients treated in periods more than 10 years before their publication of the studies. There is an impression that the prognosis in ulcerative colitis has been improving in recent years, and it will be interesting to read future reports. The physician can reassure the patient of the improving prognosis and should point out the benefits that modern medicine appears to be achieving with this condition.

REFERENCES

1. Hywel Jones J, Lennard-Jones JE, Morson BC, et al: Numerical taxonomy and discriminant analysis applied to non-specific colitis. *Q J Med* 42:715, 1973.
2. Das KM, Erber WF, Rubinstein A: Immunohistochemical changes in morphologically involved and uninvolved colonic mucosa of patients with idiopathic proctitis. *J Clin Invest* 59:379, 1977.
3. Crohn BB, Ginzburg L, Oppenheimer GD: Regional ileitis: Pathologic and clinical entity. *JAMA* 99:1323, 1932.
4. Colp R: A case of nonspecific granuloma of the terminal ileum and caecum. *Surg Clin North Am* 14:443, 1934.
5. Lockhart-Mummery HE, Morson BC: Crohn's disease (regional enteritis) of the large intestine and its distinction from ulcerative colitis. *Gut* 1:87, 1960.
6. Miller DS, Keighley AC, Smith PG, et al: Crohn's disease in Nottingham: A search for time-space clustering. *Gut* 16:454, 1975.
7. Brahme F, Lindström C, Weckert A: Crohn's disease in a defined population. *Gastroenterology* 69:342, 1975.
8. Evans JG, Acheson ED: An epidemiological study of ulcerative colitis and regional enteritis in the Oxford area. *Gut* 6:311, 1965.
9. Birnbaum D, Groen JJ, Kallner G: Ulcerative colitis among the ethnic groups of Israel. *Arch Intern Med* 105:843, 1960.
10. Bonnevie O: A socioeconomic study of patients with ulcerative colitis. *Scand J Gastroenterol* 2:129, 1967.
11. Gitnick GL, Rosen VJ: Viral investigations of inflammatory bowel disease. *Gastroenterology* 72:1062, 1977.
12. Asquith P, Mackintosh P, Stokes PL, et al: Histocompatibility antigens in patients with inflammatory bowel disease. *Lancet* 1:113, 1974.
13. Korsmeyer SJ, Williams RC, Wilson ID, et al: Lymphocytotoxic antibody in inflammatory bowel disease. *N Engl J Med* 293:1117, 1975.
14. Cave DR, Mitchell DN, Brooke BN: Evidence of an agent transmissible from ulcerative colitis tissue. *Lancet* 1:1311, 1976.
15. Cave DR, Kane SP, Mitchell DN: Further animal evidence of a transmissible agent in Crohn's disease. *Lancet* 2:1120, 1973.
16. Perlmann P, Hammarström S, Lagercrantz R, et al: Autoantibodies to colon in rats and human ulcerative colitis: Cross reactivity with *Escherichia coli* 0:14. *Proc Soc Exp Biol Med* 125:975, 1967.
17. Jewell DP, MacLennan ICM: Circulating immune complexes in inflammatory bowel disease. *Clin Exp Immunol* 14:219, 1973.
18. Perlmann P, Broberger O: *In vitro* studies of ulcerative colitis: II. Cytotoxic action of white blood cells from patients on human fetal colon cells. *J Exp Med* 117:717, 1963.

19. Heatley RV, Rhodes J, Calcraft BJ, et al: Immunoglobulin E in rectal mucosa of patients with proctitis. *Lancet* 2:1010, 1975.
20. Skinner JM, Whitehead R: The plasma cells in inflammatory disease of the colon: A quantitative study. *J Clin Pathol* 27:643, 1974.
21. Panem S, Ordóñez NG, Kirsten WH, et al: C-type virus expression in systemic lupus erythematosus. *N Engl J Med* 295:470, 1976.
22. Wright R, Truelove SC: A controlled therapeutic trial of various diets in ulcerative colitis. *Br Med J* 2:138, 1965.
23. Peña AS, Truelove SC: Hypolactasia and ulcerative colitis. *Gastroenterology* 64:400, 1973.
24. Monk M, Mendeloff AI, Siegel CI, et al: An epidemiological study of ulcerative colitis and regional enteritis among adults in Baltimore. *J Chronic Dis* 22:565, 1970.
25. Bartrop RW, Luckhurst E, Lazarus L, et al: Depressed lymphocyte function after bereavement. *Lancet* 1:834, 1977.
26. Fitterer JD, Cromwell LG, Sims JE: Colonic obstruction by giant pseudopolyps. *Gastroenterology* 72: 153, 1977.
27. Cook MG, Dixon MF: An analysis of the reliability of detection and diagnostic value of various pathological features in Crohn's disease and ulcerative colitis. *Gut* 14:255, 1973.
28. Bleiberg H, Mainguet P, Galand P, et al: Cell renewal in the human rectum: *In vitro* autoradiographic study on active ulcerative colitis. *Gastroenterology* 58:851, 1970.
29. Whitehead R: *Mucosal Biopsy of the Gastrointestinal Tract.* Philadelphia and London, WB Saunders, 1973.
30. Kwaan HC, Cocco A, Mendeloff AI, et al: Fibrinolytic activity in the normal and inflamed rectal mucosa. *Scand J Gastroenterol* 4:441, 1969.
31. Soergel KH, Ingelfinger FJ: Composition of rectal mucus in normal subjects and patients with ulcerative colitis. *Gastroenterology* 47:610, 1964.
32. MacDermott RP, Donaldson RM, Trier JS: Glycoprotein synthesis and secretion by mucosal biopsies of rabbit colon and human rectum. *J Clin Invest* 54:545, 1974.
33. Farman J, Twersky J, Fierst S: Ulcerative colitis associated with hypertrophic osteoarthropathy. *Am J Dig Dis* 21:130, 1976.
34. De Dombal FT, Watts JM, Watkinson G, et al: Local complications of ulcerative colitis: Stricture, pseudopolyposis, and carcinoma of colon and rectum. *Br Med J* 1:1442, 1966.
35. Edwards FC, Truelove SC: The course and prognosis of ulcerative colitis. *Gut* 4:299, 1963; 5:1, 1964.
36. Mallas EG, Mackintosh P, Asquith P, et al: Histocompatibility antigens in inflammatory bowel disease. *Gut* 17:906, 1976.
37. Perrett AD, Higgins G, Johnson HH, et al: The liver in ulcerative colitis. *Q J Med* 40:211, 1971.
38. Brooke BN, Slaney G: Portal bacteraemia in ulcerative colitis. *Lancet* 1:1206, 1958.
39. Ritchie JK, Allan RN, Macartney J, et al: Biliary tract carcinoma associated with ulcerative colitis. *Q J Med* 63:263, 1974.
40. Lam A, Borda IT, Inwood MJ, et al: Coagulation studies in ulcerative colitis and Crohn's disease. *Gastroenterology* 68:245, 1975.
41. Bennett RC, Hughes ESR: Urinary calculi and ulcerative colitis. *Br Med J* 2:494, 1972.

42. Goldstone AH: Autoimmune haemolytic anaemia in ulcerative colitis. *Br Med J* 2:556, 1974.
43. Pounder RE, Craven ER, Henthorn JS, et al: Red cell abnormalities associated with sulphasalazine maintenance therapy for ulcerative colitis. *Gut* 16:181, 1975.
44. Franklin JL, Rosenberg IH: Impaired folic acid absorption in inflammatory bowel disease: Effects of salicylazosulfapyridine. *Gastroenterology* 62:845, 1972.
45. Wackers FJT, Tytgat GN, Vreeken J: Necrotizing vasculitis and ulcerative colitis. *Br Med J* 4:83, 1974.
46. Kraft SC, Earle RH, Roesler M, et al: Unexplained bronchopulmonary disease with inflammatory bowel disease. *Arch Intern Med* 136:454, 1976.
47. Eade OE, Smith CL, Whorwell PJ: Pulmonary function in patients with inflammatory bowel disease. *Gut* 18:A423, 1977.
48. Jewell DP, Truelove SC: Raeginic hypersensitivity in ulcerative colitis. *Gut* 13:903, 1972.
49. Goodman MJ, Moir DJ, Holt JM, et al: Pericarditis associated with ulcerative colitis and Crohn's disease. *Am J Dig Dis* 21:98, 1976.
50. Järnerot G, Azad Khan AK, Truelove SC: The thyroid in ulcerative colitis and Crohn's disease. *Acta Med Scand* 197:83, 1975.
51. Vantrappen G, Ponette E, Geboes K, et al: *Yersinia* enteritis and enterocolitis: Gastroenterological aspects. *Gastroenterology* 72:220, 1977.
52. Rutter KRP, Riddell RH: The solitary ulcer syndrome of the rectum. *Clin Gastroenterol* 4:505, 1975.
53. Schachter H, Kirsner JB: *Crohn's Disease.* New York, John Wiley & Sons, Inc, 1978.
54. Meisel JL, Bergman D, Graney D, et al: Human rectal mucosa: Proctoscopic and morphological changes caused by laxatives. *Gastroenterology* 72:1274, 1977.
55. Truelove SC, Reynell PC: *Diseases of the Digestive System,* ed. 2. Oxford, Blackwell Scientific Publications, 1972, p. 441.
56. Bohlman TW, Katon RM, Lipshutz GR, et al: Fiberoptic pansigmoidoscopy. *Gastroenterology* 72:644, 1977.
57. Prolla JC, Kirsner JB: *Handbook and Atlas of Gastrointestinal Exfoliative Cytology.* Chicago, University of Chicago Press, 1972.
58. Crapp AR, Powis SJA, Tillotson P, et al: Preparation of the bowel by whole-gut irrigation. *Lancet* 2:1239, 1975.
59. Fielding JF, Lumsden K: Large-bowel perforations in patients undergoing sigmoidoscopy and barium enema. *Br Med J* 1:471, 1973.
60. McAlister WH, Anderson MS, Bloomberg GR, et al: Lethal effects of tannic acid in the barium enema. *Radiology* 80:765, 1963.
61. Fennessy JJ, Sparberg M, Kirsner JB: Early roentgen manifestations of mild ulcerative colitis and proctitis. *Radiology* 87:848, 1966.
62. Kirsner JB: Problems in the differentiation of ulcerative colitis and Crohn's disease of the colon: The need for repeated diagnostic evaluation. *Gastroenterology* 68:187, 1975.
63. Truelove SC, Witts LJ: Cortisone and corticotrophin in ulcerative colitis. *Br Med J* 1:387, 1959.

64. Baron JH, Connell AM, Kanaghinis TG, et al: Outpatient treatment of ulcerative colitis: Comparison between three doses of oral prednisone. *Br Med J* 2:441, 1962.
65. Truelove SC, Jewell DP: Intensive intravenous regimen for severe attacks of ulcerative colitis. *Lancet* 1:1067, 1974.
66. Truelove SC: Systemic and local corticosteroid therapy in ulcerative colitis. *Br Med J* 1:464, 1960.
67. Azad Khan AK, Truelove SC: The actions of sulphasalazine, in Truelove SC, Ritchie JA (eds): *Topics in Gastroenterology 4*. Oxford, Blackwell Scientific Publications, 1976, p. 367.
68. Dissanayake AS, Truelove SC: A controlled therapeutic trial of long-term maintenance treatment of ulcerative colitis with sulphasalazine. *Gut* 14:923, 1973.
69. Das KM, Eastwood MA, McManus JPA, et al: The metabolism of salicylazosulphapyridine in ulcerative colitis. *Gut* 14:631, 1973.
70. Baron JH, Connell AM, Lennard-Jones JE, et al: Sulphasalazine and salicylazosulphadimidine in ulcerative colitis. *Lancet* 1:1094, 1962.
71. Gould SR, Lennard-Jones JE: Production of prostaglandins in ulcerative colitis and their inhibition by sulphasalazine. *Gut* 17:828, 1976.
72. Rosenberg JL, Wall AJ, Levin B, et al: A controlled trial of azathioprine in the management of ulcerative colitis. *Gastroenterology* 69:96, 1975.
73. Jewell DP, Truelove SC: Azathioprine in ulcerative colitis: Final report on a controlled therapeutic trial. *Br Med J* 4:627, 1974.
74. Singleton JW: The National Cooperative Crohn's Disease Study: Preliminary results of Part I. *Gastroenterology* 70:938, 1976.
75. Korelitz BI, Winsch M: Long-term therapy of ulcerative colitis with 6-mercaptopurine. *Am J Dig Dis* 17:111, 1972.
76. Oberling F, Hiebel G: Intravenous antilymphocytic serum in the treatment of severe rectocolitis. *N Engl J Med* 285:410, 1971.
77. West B, Lendrum R, Hill MJ, et al: Effects of sulphasalazine on faecal flora in patients with inflammatory bowel disease. *Gut* 15:960, 1974.
78. Clark CE, Powis SJA, Crapp AR, et al: Antibiotic-induced pseudomembranous colitis. *Gut* 16:824, 1975.
79. Savidge RS: Trimethoprim and sulfamethoxazole in ulcerative colitis. *Postgrad Med J* 45 (suppl):101, 1969.
80. Heatley RV, Calcraft BJ, Rhodes J, et al: Disodium cromoglycate in the treatment of chronic proctitis. *Gut* 16:559, 1975.
81. Mani V, Lloyd G, Green FHY, et al: Treatment of ulcerative colitis with oral disodium cromoglycate. *Lancet* 1:439, 1976.
82. Dudrick SJ, MacFadyen BV, Van Buren CT, et al: Parenteral alimentation: Metabolic problems and solutions. *Ann Surg* 176:259, 1972.
83. Baron JH: Montezuma's revenge. *Lancet* 2:143, 1976.
84. McMahon AW, Schmitt P, Patterson JF, et al: Personality differences between inflammatory bowel disease patients and their healthy siblings. *Psychosom Med* 35:91, 1973.
85. Jeffery PJ, Ritchie JK, Parks AG: Treatment of haemorrhoids in patients with inflammatory bowel disease. *Lancet* 1:1084, 1977.
86. Eade MN, Cooke WT, Brooke BN: Liver disease in ulcerative colitis: II. The long-term effect of colectomy. *Ann Intern Med* 72:489, 1970.

87. Soloway RD, Summerskill WHJ, Baggenstoss AH, et al: Clinical, biochemical, and histological remission of the severe chronic active liver disease: A controlled study of treatments and early prognosis. *Gastroenterology* 63:820, 1972.
88. Morson BC, Pang LSC: Rectal biopsy as an aid to cancer control in ulcerative colitis. *Gut* 8:423, 1967.
89. Dilawari JB, Lennard-Jones JE, Mackay AM, et al: Estimation of carcinoembryonic antigen in ulcerative colitis with special reference to malignant change. *Gut* 16:255, 1975.
90. Isaacson P: Tissue demonstration of carcinoembryonic antigen in ulcerative colitis. *Gut* 17:561, 1976.
91. Jalan KN, Sircus W, Card WI, et al: An experience of ulcerative colitis: I. Toxic dilation in 55 cases. *Gastroenterology* 57:68, 1969.
92. Lee ECG, Dowling BL: Perimuscular excision of the rectum for Crohn's disease and ulcerative colitis. *Br J Surg* 59:29, 1972.
93. Brooke BN: Management of ileostomy including its complications. *Lancet* 2:102, 1952.
94. Sanders RA, Sheldon GF: Septic complications of total parenteral nutrition. *Am J Surg* 132:214, 1976.
95. Schulak JA, Moossa AR, Block GE, et al: Convulsions complicating colectomy in inflammatory bowel disease. *JAMA* 237:1456, 1977.
96. Turnbull RB, Hawk WA, Weakley FL: The surgical treatment of toxic megacolon: Ileostomy and colostomy to prepare patients for colectomy. *Am J Surg* 122:325, 1971.
97. Aylett SO: Three hundred cases of diffuse ulcerative colitis treated by total colectomy and ileorectal anastomosis. *Br Med J* 1:1001, 1966.
98. Kock NG: Ileostomy without external appliances: A survey of 25 patients provided with an intra-abdominal intestinal reservoir. *Ann Surg* 173:545, 1971.
99. Goligher JC, Lintott D: Experience with 26 reservoir ileostomies. *Br J Surg* 62:893, 1975.
100. Editorial: Magnetic device to make colostomies continent. *Br Med J* 1:1238, 1977.
101. Hampton JM: Rectal mucosal stripping: A technique for preservation of the rectum after total colectomy for chronic ulcerative colitis. *Dis Colon Rectum* 19:133, 1976.
102. Sparberg M: *The Ileostomy Case.* Springfield, Ill., Charles C. Thomas, 1971.
103. Ritchie JK: Ileostomy and excisional surgery for chronic inflammatory disease of the colon: A survey of one hospital region. *Gut* 12:528, 1971.
104. Morowitz DA, Kirsner JB: Mortality in ulcerative colitis: 1930 to 1966. *Gastroenterology* 57:481, 1969.
105. Truelove SC: Medical aspects of ulcerative colitis in childhood. *Proc R Soc Med* 66:1032, 1973.
106. De Dombal FT, Watts JM, Watkinson G, et al: Ulcerative colitis and pregnancy. *Lancet* 2:599, 1965.
107. McEwan HP: Ulcerative colitis in pregnancy. *Proc R Soc Med* 65:279, 1972.
108. Fraser EC, Fainstat TD: Production of congenital defects in the offspring of pregnant mice treated with cortisone. *Pediatrics* 8:527, 1951.

109. Warrel DW, Taylor R: Outcome for the foetus of mothers receiving prednisolone during pregnancy. *Lancet* 1:117, 1968.
110. Hudson CN: Ileostomy in pregnancy. *Proc R Soc Med* 65:281, 1972.
111. Watts JM, De Dombal FT, Watkinson G, et al: The long-term prognosis of ulcerative colitis. *Br Med J* 1:1447, 1966.
112. Jalan KN, Prescott RJ, Sircus W, et al: An experience of ulcerative colitis: II. Short term outcome; III. Long term outcome. *Gastroenterology* 59:589, 1970.
113. Lennard-Jones JE, Ritchie JK, Hilder W, et al: Assessment of severity in colitis: A preliminary study. *Gut* 16:579, 1975.
114. De Dombal FT: Prognostic value of the serum proteins during severe attacks of ulcerative colitis. *Gut* 9:144, 1968.
115. Goodman MJ, Kent PW, Truelove SC: Glucosamine synthetase activity of the colonic mucosa in ulcerative colitis and Crohn's disease. *Gut* 18:219, 1977.
116. Fawaz KA, Glotzer DJ, Goldman H, et al: Ulcerative colitis and Crohn's disease of the colon: A comparison of the long-term postoperative courses. *Gastroenterology* 71:372, 1976.
117. Correspondence: Ulcerative colitis and Crohn's disease of the colon: Their postoperative courses. *Gastroenterology* 72:775, 1977.
118. Farmer RG, Brown CH: Course and prognosis of ulcerative proctosigmoiditis. *Am J Gastroenterol* 56:227, 1971.

INDEX

Abdomen, examination, 38
  pain in, 34, 69
  X-ray, 89, 106
Abortion, therapeutic, 126, 177, 179
Abscess, intra-abdominal, 154
  liver, 58
  pelvic, 155, 156
  perianal, 49, 159
  pericolic, 18, 21, 46
    treatment, 133, 148
  subphrenic, 155
Acetaminophen, 133
Acidosis, 129
ACTH, 110, 114
Adrenal cortex, suppression, 114, 153
Adrenocorticosteroids, *see* Corticosteroids
Adrenocorticotropic hormone, *see* ACTH
Age, 8, 186
Agranulocytosis, 123
Air-contrast barium enema, 100, 146
Alcohol, 141
Alimentation, parenteral, 116, 117, 131
Alopecia, 125
Amebiasis, 24, 72, 82, 84, 103
Ampicillin, 116, 127, 135
Amyloidosis, hepatic, 58
Anal lesions, *see* Perianal complications
Anatomical distribution, 3, 16
Anemia, 61
  hemolytic, 61, 122, 130
  iron deficiency, 61, 129
  megaloblastic, 62, 123
  treatment, 129
Angiodysplasia, 69
Ankylosing spondylitis, *see* Spondylitis
Anoscopy, 78, 81
Antibiotics, 116, 126, 135, 152, 154
Anticholinergics, 45, 133
Anticoagulants, 69, 87, 142
Antidepressants, 136
Antilymphocytic serum, 126
Antispasmodics, 133
Anxiety state, 136
Aphthous stomatitis, 38, 54, 140
Appearance of patient, 37
Arthralgia, 123
Arthritis, 52, 123
  rheumatoid, 51
  treatment, 139
Atelectasis, 129
Athletic activity, 137, 167
Atopic disorders, 13, 63
Atropine, 45
Azathioprine, 118, 124, 171, 174
  for chronic active hepatitis, 141
  contraindications, 126, 140
  side effects, 125
Azulfidine, *see* Sulfasalazine

Bacteroides fragilis, 127
Bactrim, 128, 135
Balantidium coli, 24, 72, 82
Barium enema X-ray, 91
  air-contrast, 100, 146
  in children, 170
  indications, 92, 146
  postevacuation, 99
  in pregnancy, 175
Barium follow-through X-ray, 102
Barium meal X-ray, 76, 103
Bed rest, 137
Behcet's disease, 73, 103
Belladonna, 45, 133
Bellergal, 45
Betamethasone, 111
Bile duct carcinoma, 58, 185
  treatment, 141
Biochemical screen, 75, 145
Biopsy, colonoscopic, 84, 88, 147
  liver, 55, 59
  rectal, 19, 85, 93, 147, 170
    complications, 87
Bisacodyl, 133
Bladder function, postoperative, 155
Bleeding, postoperative, 154
Bleeding from colon, 31, 41, 69

biopsy causing, 87
occult, 32
treatment, 129, 149
Blood dyscrasias, 122
Blood tests, 75, 125, 145
Blood transfusion, 129
Bowel habit, 132
Bowel preparation for surgery, 152
Bowel rest, 116

Calcium, 132
Calculi, 60, 166
treatment, 142
Candidiasis, 24, 72, 82, 103, 112
Cardiac disorders, 63, 156
Carcinoembryonic antigen (CEA), 147
Carcinoma of colon, 68, 81
complicating ulcerative colitis, 23, 25, 47, 133
detection, 40, 80, 101, 146
pathology, 23, 48
precancer, 23, 147
prevention, 145, 146, 150
prognosis, 184
risk of occurrence, 48
treatment, 138, 148, 150
Cascara, 133
Cathartic colon, 27
CEA, 147
Cefazolin, 127
Cerebral complications, 60
postoperative, 156
Children, 136, 169
prognosis, 172, 190
treatment, 118, 119, 126, 170
Chloramphenicol, 116, 127
Cholangiography, percutaneous transhepatic, 59
Cholangitis, sclerosing, 57, 185
treatment, 140, 141
Cholera, 103
Cirrhosis, 58, 141, 185
Clindamycin, 26, 71, 127, 155
Clotting factors, 129
Clubbing, 38
Coagulopathies, 69, 129
Cobblestone mucosa, 83, 104
Codeine, 44, 133, 135, 166
Colace, 133
Colectomy, 148
in children, 172
partial, 158
subtotal, 157, 177
in toxic dilatation, 157
Coliform bacteria, 127
Colitis, forms of, 23, 70, 82
Colitis cystica profunda, 27
Colonoscopy, 47, 83, 147, 176
with polypectomy, 138
Colostomy, 158
Competitive activities, 137
Complications, local, 41, 80, 184
treatment, 138, 159
systemic, 50
Conjunctivitis, 54, 128, 140
Constipation, 34, 132
Contraception, 178
Contraceptive pill, 71, 135, 137, 178
Cortenema, 119
Corticosteroids, 36, 45, 110, 170, 171, 187
alternate-day, 118, 171
contraindications, 113
enemas, 119
enteric-coated, 112
foam, 121
intravenous, 116
long-term, 117
postoperative, 153
preoperative, 153
side effects, 111, 175
for side effects of sulfasalazine, 122
suppositories, 121
topical, 119
Corticotropin, 110, 114
Corticotropin-releasing hormone (CRH), 114
Cortifoam, 121
Cortisol, *see* Hydrocortisone
Cotrimoxazole, 128, 135
Crohn's disease, 73, 104
distinction from ulcerative colitis, 6, 13, 25, 83, 84, 102, 104
incidence, 7
relationship to ulcerative colitis, 4, 9, 12, 13
Cromoglycate, disodium, *see* Cromolyn
Cromolyn, 128, 171, 175
Crypt abscess, 20
Crypt distortion, 20
Crypt hypertrophy, 21
Cutaneous manifestations, *see* Skin lesions
Cytology, 88

Darvon, 133
Death, causes of, 189
mortality rate, 187
Definition, 3, 6
Dehydration, 38, 129
Demerol, 44, 133
Depression, 36, 113, 136
Dermatitis, exfoliative, 122
Dexamethasone, 111
DF-118, 45, 135
Diabetes mellitus, 114
Diagnosis, 3, 67
differential, 23, 67, 81, 103
Dialose, 133
Diameter of colon, 91
Diarrhea, 32, 68, 80
travelers', 135
treatment, 132, 150
Diazepam, 133

Diet, 117, 129, 134
bland, 134
elemental, 130
for ileostomy patient, 164
postoperative, 153
Dihydrocodeine, 45, 135
Dilatation, toxic, 18, 25, 42, 90, 187
barium enema leading to, 43, 45
drug-induced, 44, 133
prevention, 44
treatment, 44, 109, 117, 149
Dioctyl-Medo, 133
Dioctyl sodium sulfosuccinate, 133
Diphenoxylate, 45, 132
Disodium cromoglycate, *see* Cromolyn
Distalgesic, 133
Diverticulitis, 68, 81
Diverticulosis, 68, 103
Donnatal, 45
Dysentery, amebic, 24, 72, 82, 84, 103
bacillary, 24, 70, 82, 103
Dysplasia, epithelial, 22, 84, 147, 149

Edema, 112
Effersyllium, 133
Electrocardiography, 75, 152
Electrolytes, 36, 112, 129, 132, 152, 165
Embolism, air, 132
mesenteric, 72
pulmonary, 60, 63, 129, 141, 156
Emotional factors, 14, 136
Endometriosis, 81
Endoscopic retrograde cholangiopancreatography (ERCP), 59
Endoscopy, 77
Enema, barium, *see* Barium enema X-ray
corticosteroid, 119
preparation for sigmoidoscopy, 78
sulfasalazine, 124
Ensure, 130
Enteritis, regional, *see* Crohn's disease
Epidemiology, 6
Epilepsy, 156
Episcleritis, 55, 140
Epithelial dysplasia, 22, 84, 147, 149
Epsilon-aminocaproic acid, 32
ERCP, 59
Erythema nodosum, 52, 122, 140
Erythromycin, 135
Escherichia coli, antibody to 0:14, 12
toxigenic, 70, 82, 103, 135
Estrogens, 135, 137
Etiology, 11
Evaluation of patient, 75
Exercise, 137
Exfoliative cytology, 88
Extent of bowel involvement, 3, 16, 184
Extracolonic manifestations, 13, 16, 40, 50, 76
prognosis, 184
radiology, 105
treatment, 139, 150
Eye lesions, 54
treatment, 140

Factitious proctitis, 74
Factor VIII, 129
Familial occurrence, 9, 11, 136
Ferrous fumarate, 130
Ferrous gluconate, 130
Fetus, 174
Fever, 37, 187
Fiberoptic sigmoidoscopy, 84
Fibrinolytic activity, 32
Fissures, perianal, 23, 49, 81
treatment, 159
Fistulae, perianal, 23, 49, 81
treatment, 159
Flagyl, 128
Fluid replacement, 132, 153, 165
Foam, corticosteroid, 121
Folic acid, 62, 130
Follow-through, barium, 102
Follow-up, 144
Fortral, 44, 133
Fulminant ulcerative colitis, 41, 76, 92

Gallstones, 58, 141
Gases, blood, 129
Gastroenteritis, 70, 71, 103, 135
in ileostomy patient, 166
Gastrointestinal X-ray series, lower, *see* Barium enema X-ray
small bowel, 102
upper, *see* Barium meal X-ray
Genetics, 9, 11
Gentamicin, 127, 155
Geographical factors, 9, 136
Germinal cells, damage to, 125, 126
Giardia lamblia, 72, 82, 136
Globulins, serum, 187
Glucagon, 94
Glucocorticoids, 111
Glucosamine synthetase, 187
Glucose-6-phosphate dehydrogenase deficiency, 122
Goblet cell depletion, 20
Gonococcal proctitis, 72, 82, 103
Granulomatous colitis, *see* Crohn's disease
Growth retardation, 36, 118, 171

Headache, 123
Heinz body formation, 122
Hematocrit, 75, 129, 130, 145
Hematological parameters, 75, 125, 145
Hemoglobin, 75, 129, 130, 145, 152
Hemolysis, 61, 122, 130
Hemorrhage, *see* Bleeding

Hemorrhage from colon, *see* Bleeding from colon
Hemorrhagic disorders, 69, 129
Hemorrhagic proctitis, 4, 7
Hemorrhoids, 68, 81, 103
  treatment, 139, 159
Hepatitis, 55, 185
  chronic active, 57, 140, 141, 185
Hepatobiliary complications, 55, 185
  diagnosis, 59
  treatment, 140
Heredity, 9
Hernia, internal, 155, 178
  para-ileostomy, 155
Histocompatibility antigens, 11, 51
Histoplasmosis, 24, 72, 82, 103
Hospitalization, 110, 136
Hydrocortisone, 110
  enemas, 119
  suppositories, 121
Hydrophilic colloids, 133
Hyoscine, 45
Hyperalimentation, parenteral, 117, 131, 152, 171
  complications, 132
Hyperglycemia, 132
Hypertension, 114
  benign intracranial, 60
Hypertrophy, crypt, 21
  muscularis mucosae, 21
Hypoalbuminemia, 36, 112, 152, 187
Hypocalcemia, 132
Hypolactasia, 14, 69, 130, 134, 136
Hypomagnesemia, 132
Hypotension, 127
Hypoxia, 129

Ileitis, backwash, 4, 16, 97, 103
  prestomal, 155
  regional, *see* Crohn's disease
Ileocolitis, *see* Crohn's disease
Ileorectal anastomosis, 157, 189
Ileostomy, 150, 160, 183
  appliances, 160
  care of, 160
  in children, 172
  complications, 155, 163
  continent, 159, 189
  fluid loss, 165
  odor, 167
  patients' associations, 160
  patient's equipment, 160
  in pregnancy, 177
  prognosis, 167, 188
  prolapse, 165, 177
  psychological problems, 167
  retraction, 165
  social problems, 167
  temporary, 158, 177
  in toxic dilatation, 157
Ileus, postoperative, 184
Immune complexes, 12, 13
Immunohistochemistry, 13
Immunology, 12
Immunosuppressive agents, 124
Imodium, 45, 133, 166
Imuran, *see* Azathioprine
Incidence, 7
Infection, postoperative, 154
Infectious agent, 11
Inflammatory bowel disease, 13
Intralipid, 131
Investigations, clinical, 75, 145
Iritis, 54
  treatment, 140
Iron, deficiency, 61, 129
  preparations, 129, 135, 175
Irritable bowel syndrome, *see* Irritable colon syndrome
Irritable colon syndrome, 68, 82, 103
  distinction from ulcerative colitis, 6, 14, 16, 27, 33, 82, 136
Ischemic colitis, 25, 71, 82, 84, 103
Iso-Gel, 133

Jaundice, 57, 58
Jews, 9
Joint disorders, 51, 123, 139

Kidney disorders, 60, 142, 166

Laxatives, 133
  abuse, 82, 103
  preparation for barium enema X-ray, 93
  prior to sigmoidoscopy, 78
Leukemic involvement of rectum, 69, 82, 103
Leukocytosis, 113
Life expectancy, 183
Lincomycin, 26, 71
Liver, fatty, 55, 132, 141
Liver abscess, 58
Liver biopsy, 55, 59
Liver disease, 55, 140
  drug-induced, 59
  use of azathioprine, 125
Liver function tests, 59, 75, 146
Lomotil, 45, 132, 166
Loperamide, 45, 133, 166
Lymphocytotoxic antibody, 11
Lymphogranuloma venereum, 24, 72, 82, 103
Lymphoid aggregates, 21
Lymphomatous involvement of rectum, 69, 82, 103

Macroscopic appearances, 16
Magnesium, 132
Magnetic stoma devices, 159
Malabsorption, 34
Malnutrition, 129, 131, 171

Marrow suppression, 62, 125
Mass, abdominal, 39
Medical treatment, *see* Treatment, medical
Medrol, *see* Methylprednisolone
Medrol En-Pak, 119
Megacolon, toxic, *see* Dilatation, toxic
Melanosis coli, 82
Membranous colitis, 26, 71, 82, 103
Meperidine, 44, 133
6-Mercaptopurine, 126
Mesenteric vascular disease, 71
Metamucil, 133
Methylcellulose, 133
Methylprednisolone, 111, 116
  topical, 119
Metronidazole, 128
Microscopic appearances, 18
Mild ulcerative colitis, 76, 81, 191
  treatment, 121, 129
Milk, 14, 134
Mineral elements, 132
Moderate ulcerative colitis, 76, 81
  treatment, 115, 121, 129
Morphine, 44
Mortality, 187
Mouth, 38, 54, 140
"Mucous colitis," 6
Mucus, in crypts, 21
  in stools, 33
Munchausen syndrome, 74
Myocarditis, 63, 129, 143

Nalcrom, *see* Cromolyn
Nausea, due to sulfasalazine, 122
Nephrolithiasis, 60, 142, 166
Normacol Special, 133
Nutrition, 129
  restoration of, 130

Obesity, 167
Obstruction, intestinal, 155, 163, 178
Ocular complications, *see* Eye lesions
Opiates, 44, 133, 135
Orange-colored urine, 123
Osteoarthropathy, hypertrophic, 38
Osteoporosis, 112, 114

Pain, abdominal, 34, 69
  postprandial, 35
  rectal, 35
  treatment, 133, 150
Pancreatitis, 125
Paneth cell metaplasia, 21
Paracetamol, 133
Paraffin, 133
Paratyphoid, 71, 82
Parenteral feeding, *see* Alimentation, parenteral
Parents, 15, 136, 170, 172
Pathilon, 45
Pathology, 16
Pelvic examination, 40
Penicillin, 127, 135
Pentazocine, 44, 133
Peptic ulceration, 114
Perforation, 18, 21, 45, 91
  biopsy causing, 87
  "silent," 45
  treatment, 126, 148
Perianal complications, 23, 49
  treatment, 138, 159
Pericarditis, 63, 129
Pericholangitis, 55
  treatment, 140
Perimuscular excision of rectum, 150
Peripheral manifestations, *see* Extracolonic manifestations
Peritonitis, 21, 45, 46
  postoperative, 154
  treatment, 133, 148
Pethidine, 44, 133
pH, arterial, 129
Phenobarbital, 133
Phenoxybenzamine, 32
Photosensitivity, 122
Phthalylsulfathiazole, 127
Physical signs, 37
Physician, role of, 4, 144
Pneumothorax, 132
Polyps, 17
  adenomatous, 23, 40, 69, 81, 138
Postevacuation barium enema, 99
Postoperative care, 152
Potassium, 36, 112, 128, 152, 165
Precision Isotonic, 130
Prednisolone, 111
  enemas, 119
  eyedrops, 140
  suppositories, 121
Prednisolone-21-phosphate, 116
Prednisolone sodium succinate, 116
Prednisone, 111
  for hepatic complications, 141
Predsol Retention Enemas, 119
Pregnancy, 126, 137, 173, 186
  avoidance, 178
  termination, 126, 177, 179
Preoperative care, 152
Presacral space, 95
Prevalence, 7
Prevention, 134
  of relapse, 118, 121, 134
Pro-Banthine, 45, 133
Proctitis, hemorrhagic, 4, 7
  idiopathic, 4
  ulcerative, 4, 7, 81
    treatment, 120, 121
Proctocolectomy, 150
  complications, 153

two-stage, 157
Proctoscopy, 78
Progestogens, 135, 137
Prognosis, 183
Prolapse, ileostomy, 165, 177
rectal, 82
Propantheline bromide, 45, 133, 135
Propoxyphene, 133
Protein repletion, 129, 152
Prothrombin, time, 129
Pruritus, 57
ani, 139
Pseudomembranous colitis, *see* Membranous colitis
Pseudopolyps, 17, 23, 25, 40, 46, 80, 84, 98, 100, 101
Psychiatrically-disturbed patient, 114
Psychological changes due to steroid therapy, 113
Psychological factors, 14, 136
in children, 170
Psychological problems of ileostomy patient, 167
Psychotherapy, 136
Psyllium, 133
Puerperium, 173, 186
Pulmonary disorders, 63, 123
postoperative, 156
Pulmonary embolism, 60, 63, 129, 141, 156
Pulmonary function tests, 152
Pulmonary infiltration, 63, 123, 129
Purgatives, *see* Laxatives
Pus in stools, 33
Pyoderma gangrenosum, 53
treatment, 140

Quiescent ulcerative colitis, 76, 81
treatment, 121

Race, 9
Radiation colitis, 26, 72, 82, 104
Radiation enteritis, 73
Radiation proctitis, 73, 82, 104
Radiology, 89
in pregnancy, 175
Rectal bleeding, *see* Bleeding from colon
Rectal examination, 39
Rectal mucosal stripping, 159
Rectal sparing, 16, 84, 96
Rectal ulcer, solitary, 26, 73, 83
Rectomucous fistula, 157, 177
Rehydration, 129
Relapse, prevention, 118, 121, 134
rate, 191
Renal complications, 60, 142, 166
Rest, 136
Resuscitation, 128
Reticulum cell sarcoma, 125
Retrorectal space, 95
Rodney Smith tube, 141
Rotaviruses, 70
Roughage, 134

Sacroiliitis, 51, 105
treatment, 139
Salazopyrin, *see* Sulfasalazine
Salicylazosulfapyridine, *see* Sulfasalazine
Salmonella, 71, 82, 103
Schistosomiasis, 24, 72
Senna, 133
Septicemia, 126, 129
Septra, 128, 135
Septrin, 128, 135
Serosal inflammation, 18, 21
Serration, 96
Severe ulcerative colitis, 76, 81, 187
barium enema during, 93
treatment, 116, 121, 128
Severity of ulcerative colitis, 76, 81, 184
false assessment, 113
Sex incidence, 8
Sexual function, 150, 156, 168
Shigella, 24, 70, 82, 103
Shock, 127, 129
Sigmoidoscopy, 77, 145
in children, 170
fiberoptic, 84
indications, 77, 145
in pregnancy, 176
prior to barium enema, 93
Signs, physical, 37
Skin lesions, 52
drug-induced, 122, 125
treatment, 140
Small bowel X-ray series, 102
Social problems of ileostomy patient, 167
Social status, 9
Sodium, 36, 112, 128, 165
Solitary rectal ulcer syndrome, 26, 73, 83
"Spastic colitis," 6
Spleen, 39
Spondylitis, ankylosing, 51, 105
treatment, 140
Sport, 137, 167
Staphylococcal enterocolitis, 26, 71
Stenosis, rectal, 80
Steroids, *see* Corticosteroids
Stomatitis, 38, 54, 140
Stool, culture, 75
microscopy, 75
Streptomycin, 127
Stress, 114, 136
Strictures, colonic, 17, 41, 81, 99, 102
treatment, 138, 149, 150
rectal, 47, 80
Suicide, 168, 190
Sulfasalazine, 121, 127, 187
in children, 170
enemas, 124
in pregnancy, 175

side effects, 61, 122
Sulfathalidine, 127
Sulfonamides, 121, 127
Suppositories, steroid, 121
Surfak, 133
Surgery, 148
in children, 172
indications, 109, 117, 118, 148
mortality, 188
in pregnancy, 176
Survival rates, 190
Symptomatic therapy, 132
Symptoms, 31

Talwin, 44, 133
Tannic acid, 94
Tenesmus, 35
Tetracycline, 116, 127
Thrombocytopenia, 123
Thromboembolism, 60, 63, 132, 156
treatment, 141
Thromboplastin time, partial, 129
"Thumbprint" ulcers, 103
Thyroid gland, 63
Topical steroids, 119
Toxic dilatation, *see* Dilatation, toxic
Tranquillizers, 133, 136
Transmissibility, 12
Traumatic rectal ulcers, 74
Travel, 136
Travelers' diarrhea, 135
Treatment, 109
of children, 170
comparison of medical and surgical, 189
failure of medical, 149
influence on prognosis, 187
medical, 109
in pregnancy, 176
surgical, 109, 148, 172, 176

Triaditis, portal, 55
Triamcinolone, 111
Trimethoprim, 128, 135
Tuberculosis, 24, 72, 82, 103
complicating steroid therapy, 112
Tylenol, 45, 133
Typhoid, 71, 82

Ulcerative proctitis, *see* Proctitis, ulcerative
Ultrasonography, 59
Urgency of stool, 33, 34
Urinalysis, 75, 145
Urinary calculi, 60, 142, 166
Urinary tract infection, postoperative, 155
Urogenital complications of colectomy, 155
Uveitis, 54

Vaginal examination, 40
Valium, 133
Vasculitis, 62, 71
Venous pressure, central, 129
Venous thrombosis, 60, 156
treatment, 141
Viral-like particles, 12
Vitamin B_{12}, 62, 130
Vitamins, 129, 130, 132
Vivonex, 130
Vomiting, due to sulfasalazine, 122

Weakness, 36
Weight loss, 35
Work, 137, 167
Wound, abdominal, 154
perineal, 154

X-rays, *see* Radiology

Yersinia enterocolitica, 71
Young patients, 118, 126